Preventing and Treating Missing Data in Longitudinal Clinical Trials

A Practical Guide

Recent decades have brought advances in statistical theory for missing data, which, combined with advances in computing ability, have allowed implementation of a wide array of analyses. In fact, so many methods are available that it can be difficult to ascertain when to use which method. This book focuses on the prevention and treatment of missing data in longitudinal clinical trials. Based on his extensive experience with missing data, the author offers advice on choosing analysis methods and on ways to prevent missing data through appropriate trial design and conduct. He offers a practical guide to key principles and explains analytic methods for the non-statistician using limited statistical notation and jargon. The book's goal is to present a comprehensive strategy for preventing and treating missing data, and to make available the programs used to conduct the analyses of the example dataset.

Craig H. Mallinckrodt is Research Fellow in the Decision Sciences and Strategy Group at Eli Lilly and Company. Dr. Mallinckrodt has supported drug development in all four clinical phases and in several therapeutic areas. He currently leads Lilly's Advanced Analytics hub for missing data and their Placebo Response Task Force, and is a member of a number of other scientific work groups. He has authored more than 170 papers, book chapters, and texts, including extensive works on missing data and longitudinal data analysis in journals such as *Statistics in Medicine*, *Pharmaceutical Statistics*, the *Journal of Biopharmaceutical Statistics*, the *Journal of Psychiatric Research*, the *Archives of General Psychiatry*, and *Nature*. He currently chairs the Drug Information Association's Scientific Working Group on Missing Data.

Practical Guides to Biostatistics and Epidemiology

Series advisors

Susan Ellenberg, *University of Pennsylvania School of Medicine*
Robert C. Elston, *Case Western Reserve University School of Medicine*
Brian Everitt, *Institute for Psychiatry, King's College London*
Frank Harrell, *Vanderbilt University Medical Center, Tennessee*
Jos W. R. Twisk, *VU University Medical Center, Amsterdam*

This series of short and practical but authoritative books is for biomedical researchers, clinical investigators, public health researchers, epidemiologists, and non-academic and consulting biostatisticians who work with data from biomedical, epidemiological, and genetic studies. Some books explore a modern statistical method and its applications, others may focus on a particular disease or condition and the statistical techniques most commonly used in studying it.

The series is for people who use statistics to answer specific research questions. Books will explain the application of techniques, specifically the use of computational tools, and emphasize the interpretation of results, not the underlying mathematical and statistical theory.

Published in the series

Applied Multilevel Analysis, by **Jos W. R. Twisk**
Secondary Data Sources for Public Health, by **Sarah Boslaugh**
Survival Analysis for Epidemiologic and Medical Research, by **Steve Selvin**
Statistical Learning for Biomedical Data, by **James D. Malley, Karen G. Malley,** and **Sinisa Pajevic**
Measurement in Medicine, by **Henrica C.W. deVet, Caroline B. Terwee, Lidwine B. Mokkink, and Dirk L. Knol**
Genomic Clinical Trials and Predictive Medicine, by **Richard M. Simon**

Preventing and Treating Missing Data in Longitudinal Clinical Trials

A Practical Guide

Craig H. Mallinckrodt

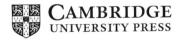

CAMBRIDGE
UNIVERSITY PRESS

CAMBRIDGE UNIVERSITY PRESS
Cambridge, New York, Melbourne, Madrid, Cape Town,
Singapore, São Paulo, Delhi, Mexico City

Cambridge University Press
32 Avenue of the Americas, New York, NY 10013-2473, USA

www.cambridge.org
Information on this title: www.cambridge.org/9781107679153

First published 2013

Printed in the United States of America

A catalog record for this publication is available from the British Library.

Library of Congress Cataloging in Publication Data

Mallinckrodt, Craig, 1958–
Preventing and treating missing data in longitudinal clinical trials:
A practical guide / Craig Mallinckrodt.
   pages cm – (Practical guides to biostatistics and epidemiology)
Includes bibliographical references and index.
ISBN 978-1-107-03138-8 (hardback) – ISBN 978-1-107-67915-3 (paperback)
1. Clinical trials – Longitudinal studies.   2. Medical sciences – Statistical methods.
3. Regression analysis – Data processing.   I. Title.
R853.C55M3374   2013
610.72′4–dc23   2012038442

ISBN 978-1-107-03138-8 Hardback
ISBN 978-1-107-67915-3 Paperback

Contents

List of Figures

List of Tables

Acknowledgments

It has been my good fortune to collaborate with many excellent researchers in the field of missing data. These collaborations were of great benefit to this book. First, many thanks to those who were forced to read early versions of this book and provided valuable feedback: Geert Molenberghs (Universiteit Hasselt, Diepenbeek), Lei Xu (Eli Lilly, Indianapolis), and Adam Meyers (BioGen Idec, Boston).

For assistance in developing the programs used to analyze example data: Ilya Lipkovich (Quintiles, Indianapolis), Hank Wei (Eli Lilly, Indianapolis), Qun Lin (Eli Lilly, Indianapolis), and Dustin Ruff (Eli Lilly, Indianapolis).

For collaborations over the years that significantly influenced the content of this book: Caroline Beunckens (Universiteit Hasselt, Diepenbeek), James Carpenter (London School of Hygiene and Tropical Medicine), Raymond Carroll (Texas A&M University, College Station), Christy Chuang-Stein (Pfizer, New York), Scott Clark (Eli Lilly, Indianapolis), Mike Detke (MedAvante, Hamilton), Ivy Jansen (Universiteit Hasselt, Diepenbeek), Chris Kaiser (Eli Lilly, Indianapolis), Mike Kenward (London School of Hygiene and Tropical Medicine), Peter Lane (Glaxosmithkline, Harlow), Andy Leon (Weill Medical College, Cornell, New York), Stacy Lindborg (BioGen Idec, Boston), Rod Little (University of Michigan, Ann Arbor), James Roger (London School of Hygiene and Tropical Medicine), Steve Ruberg (Eli Lilly, Indianapolis), Shuyi Shen (Genentech, Ocenside), Cristina Sotto (Universiteit Hasselt, Diepenbeek), Birhanu Teshome (Universiteit Hasselt, Diepenbeek),

Herbert Thijs (Universiteit Hasselt, Diepenbeek), and Russ Wolfinger (SAS, Cary).

To Donna and Marissa, for your understanding and for helping make the time possible to work on this book, and for the encouragement and support needed to finish it!

Preface

This book focuses on the prevention and treatment of missing data in longitudinal clinical trials with repeated measures, such as are common in later phases of medical research and drug development. Recent decades have brought advances in statistical theory, which, combined with advances in computing ability, have allowed implementation of a wide array of analyses. In fact, so many methods are available that it can be difficult to ascertain when to use which method. A danger in such circumstances is to blindly use newer methods without proper understanding of their strengths and limitations, or to disregard all newer methods in favor of familiar approaches.

Moreover, the complex discussions on how to analyze incomplete data have overshadowed discussions on ways to prevent missing data, which would of course be the preferred solution. Therefore, preventing missing data through appropriate trial design and conduct is given significant attention in this book. Nevertheless, despite all efforts at prevention, missing data will remain an ever-present problem and analytic approaches will continue to be an important consideration.

Recent research has fostered an emerging consensus regarding the analysis of incomplete longitudinal data. Key principles and analytic methods are explained in terms non-statisticians can understand. Although the use of equations, symbols, and Greek letters to describe the analyses is largely avoided, sufficient technical detail is provided so readers can take away more than a peripheral understanding of the methods and issues. For those with in-depth statistical interests, reference to more technical literature is provided.

Part I begins with illustrations of how missing data erode the reliability and credibility of medical research. Subsequent chapters discuss missing data mechanisms and the estimands (what is to be estimated) of interest in longitudinal trials with incomplete data. Part II covers trial design and conduct features that can help prevent missing data. Part III includes chapters on common methods of estimation, data and modeling considerations, and means of dealing with missing data (e.g., imputation). Part IV ties together the topics covered in Part III to illustrate various analyses applicable to incomplete longitudinal data. Small example data sets are used to illustrate and explain key analyses. An actual clinical trial data set is the focal point for proposing and implementing an overall analytic strategy that includes sensitivity analyses for assessing the impact of missing data.

This strategy is referred to as the analytic road map. A road map is different from driving instructions. Unlike driving directions, a road map does not chart a specific course, with instructions on exactly how far to go and when to turn. Instead, the road map lays out the alternatives so that the best route for a particular situation can be chosen.

The concluding chapter refocuses on the key issues covered throughout the book, presents a comprehensive strategy for preventing and treating missing data, and makes available the programs used to conduct the analyses of the example dataset.

Part I

BACKGROUND AND SETTING

This section begins with a chapter illustrating how missing data can cloud inferences to be drawn from clinical trials – in other words, why missing data matter. Chapter 2 focuses on the mechanisms that give rise to missing data. Understanding these mechanisms is the essential background needed to understand the possible consequences of missing data. Chapter 3 discusses estimands – what is to be estimated from the trial. Together, these chapters form the basis for discussion on how to limit missing data and how to handle missing data that remains.

Why Missing Data Matter

The evidence to support new medicines, devices, or other medical interventions is based primarily on randomized clinical trials. Many of these trials involve assessments taken at the start of treatment (baseline), followed by assessments taken repeatedly during and in some scenarios after the treatment period. In some cases, such as cancer trials, the primary post-baseline assessments are whether or not some important event occurred during the assessment intervals. These outcomes can be summarized by expressing the multiple post-baseline outcomes as a time to an event, or as a percentage of patients experiencing the event at or before some landmark time point. Alternatively, the multiple post-baseline assessments can all be used in a longitudinal, repeated measures analysis, which can either focus on a landmark time point or consider outcomes across time points.

Regardless of the specific scenario, randomization facilitates fair comparisons between treatment and control groups by balancing known and unknown factors across the groups. The intent of randomization in particular, and the design of clinical trials in general, is that differences observed between the treatment and control groups are attributable to causal differences in the treatments and not to other factors.

Missing data is an ever-present problem in clinical trials and has been the subject of considerable debate and research. In fact, the U.S. Food and Drug Administration convened an expert panel to make recommendations for the prevention and treatment of missing data (NRC, 2010). The fundamental problem caused by missing data is that the balance provided by randomization is lost if, as is usually the case, the patients who discontinue the study differ in regards to the outcome of interest from those who complete the study. This imbalance can lead to biases in the comparison of the treatment groups. As the proportion of missing data increases, the potential for greater bias increases. These biases cannot be overcome by larger sample sizes. In fact, biased results from larger studies can be even more problematic because the larger studies engender greater confidence – in the wrong result.

Missing data may arise in many ways. Intermittent missing data occurs when patients miss a scheduled assessment but attend a subsequent visit. Dropout (withdrawal, attrition) is when patients miss all subsequent assessments after a certain visit. In some trials, when patients are withdrawn from their randomly assigned treatment, no more assessments are taken. In other trials, follow-up assessments may continue. All these settings may lead to missing data, although the statistical approaches appropriate for each setting may vary.

The ICH E9 guideline (www.ich.org/cache/compo/276–254-1.html), which provides the fundamental principles that guide researchers and regulators in medical research, states that despite missing data, a trial may still be valid provided the statistical methods used are sensible. Carpenter and Kenward (2007) define a sensible analysis as one where:

1) The variation between the intervention effect estimated from the trial and that in the population is random. In other words, trial results are not systematically biased.
2) As the sample size increases, the variation between the intervention effect estimated from the trial and that in the population gets smaller and smaller. In other words, as the size of the trial increases, the estimated intervention effect hones in on the true value in the population. Such estimates are called consistent in statistical terminology.
3) The estimate of the variability between the trial intervention effect and the true effect in the population (i.e., the standard error) correctly reflects the uncertainty in the data.

If all these conditions hold, then valid inference can be drawn despite the missing data. However, the analyses required to meet these conditions may be different from the analyses that satisfy these conditions when no data are missing. Regardless, whenever data intended to be collected are missing, information is lost and estimates are less precise than if data were complete.

Table 1.1. *Hypothetical Trial Results*

	Treatment 1	Treatment 2
Success	56	42
Failure	84	98
Missing	60	60
Total	200	200

The following hypothetical data illustrates the ambiguity missing data can cause. Assume Treatment 1 is an investigational intervention or medicine and Treatment 2 is the standard of care. Results for each patient are categorized as success or failure and the outcomes are summarized in Table 1.1.

The success rates based on the observed data are 40% (56/140) for Treatment 1 and 30% (42/140) for Treatment 2. When basing results on only the patients with known outcomes, the success rates are not significantly different (p = .103). However, 30% of the outcomes are missing. Table 1.2 summarizes results that would be seen if:

1) It was assumed presence or absence of the observations was not related to the outcome. Hence, in each treatment group unknown outcomes were assumed to have the same proportion of successes as the known outcomes.
2) It was assumed all patients with unknown outcomes were failures.
3) It was assumed unknown outcomes for the investigational drug (Treatment 1) were failures, and unknown outcomes for the standard of care (Treatment 2) had an equal chance of success or failure (50% success).

Table 1.2. *Hypothetical Trial Results Under Different Assumptions About the Missing Outcomes*

	Assumption 1		Assumption 2		Assumption 3	
	Treatment 1	Treatment 2	Treatment 1	Treatment 2	Treatment 1	Treatment 2
Success	80	60	56	42	56	72
Failure	120	140	144	158	144	128

Using assumption 1, results significantly (p = .046) favored Treatment 1 because of the increase in sample size – even though the percentages of success and failure did not change compared with the results in Table 1.1. Using assumption 2, results were trending to favor Treatment 1, but the difference was not significant (p = .130). Using assumption 3, results approached significance (p = .108) in favor of Treatment 2.

These results illustrate how missing outcomes limit the extent to which the trial can inform clinical practice. According to some assumptions the success rate for Treatment 1 was significantly better than Treatment 2, but under other assumptions Treatment 2 was favored. These results also provide the motivation for trial sponsors to limit the amount of missing data. The same rates of success led to non-significance with the missing observations, but would have been significant if no data were missing (assumption 1).

Given the wide range of conclusions that may be drawn based on differing assumptions about the missing data, it may seem that trials with nontrivial amounts of missing data are uninterpretable. With missing data, some information is irretrievably lost, but disregarding the 140 observed outcomes per treatment because 60 outcomes were missing is not an answer.

The extent to which useful information can be gleaned from trials with missing data depends on the amount of missing data, how well the reasons or mechanisms driving the missingness are understood, and how robust conclusions are across the plausible reasons (mechanisms).

Although it is impossible to know with certainty what mechanisms gave rise to the missing data, the extent to which it is understood why data are missing narrows the possibilities. Results can be compared across these various possibilities. Of course, all else equal, the more complete the data the more interpretable the findings.

The importance of reducing missing data and the bias from it is further illustrated in Figure 1.1. This graph depicts the power from the contrast between drug and control from 10,000 simulated clinical trials under three assumptions. In all scenarios the true treatment effect was equal to a standardized effect size (Cohen's D) (Cohen, 1992) of 0.50, and 200 patients were randomized to drug versus control in a 1:1 ratio. The ideal scenario had only 5% dropout and no bias from it. The medium

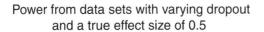

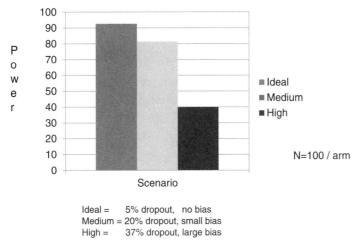

Power from data sets with varying dropout
and a true effect size of 0.5

Ideal =   5% dropout,   no bias
Medium = 20% dropout, small bias
High =   37% dropout, large bias

Figure 1.1. Power for the contrast between drug and control from 10,000 simulated clinical trials with low, medium, and high rates of dropout.

scenario had a moderate dropout rate of 20% and minimal bias as the average estimated treatment effect was 0.45, a bit smaller than the true value of 0.50. The high scenario had 40% dropout and appreciable bias as the average estimated treatment effect was only 0.30.

When using a p value of 0.05 as the cutoff for statistical significance, the ideal scenario had 92% power, the moderate scenario had 81% power, and the high dropout scenario had 40% power. In other words, moderate dropout more than doubled (8% vs. 19%) the rate of false negative findings. In the high-dropout scenario, power was reduced to only about 40%, more than doubling the false negative rate over that found with moderate dropout. Dropout can turn a study with a very high probability of success into something less sure than a coin flip.

Modern statistical analyses can reduce the potential for bias arising from missing data. However, principled means of handling missing data rely on untestable assumptions about the missing values and the mechanism giving rise to them (Verbeke and Molenberghs, 2000). The conundrum inherent to analyses of incomplete data is that data about which the missing data assumptions are made are missing. Hence, the assumptions cannot be tested from data, and the appropriateness of analyses and inference cannot be assured. The greater the rate of missing data, the greater the potential for increased bias. Therefore, minimizing missing data is the best way of dealing with it (Fleming, 2011).

Research on the merits of various analytic approaches for incomplete data includes literally hundreds of scenarios and millions of data sets. Comparing analytic methods can be done using simulated data with known values of the parameters being estimated. Various analytic approaches can be compared within each simulated data set or within each actual clinical trial data set. Hence, much is known about the comparative merits of analytic approaches. Parts III and IV discuss and illustrate some of the common analytic approaches.

A useful by-product of the debates on the appropriateness of various analytic approaches has been consideration of the primary estimand – that is, the primary research question in the clinical trial (see Chapter 3). Obviously, what is being estimated can influence the best way to estimate it. Determining the primary estimand is more complicated than simply stating the primary analysis. Further consideration must be given to a variety of issues. For example, should data after initiation of rescue medications and/or discontinuation of initially randomized study medication be included in the primary analysis?

Sensitivity analyses are a series of analyses with differing assumptions. The aim is that by comparing results across sensitivity analyses it becomes apparent how much inference about the treatment effect relies on the assumptions. In fact, many of the newer statistical approaches are finding their best application as sensitivity analyses rather than as a primary means of analysis (Molenberghs and Kenward, 2007; Mallinckrodt et al., 2008; NRC, 2010; also see section 12.4).

Reasonable measures to reduce missing data combined with appropriate analytic plans that include sensitivity analyses can markedly reduce the uncertainty in results and increase the information gained from medical research. Recent research has provided useful guidance on these various approaches, and the intent of this book is to provide researchers with a practical guide to make use of them.

Missing Data Mechanisms

2.1 Introduction

One of the keys to understanding the potential impact of missing data is to understand the mechanism(s) that gave rise to the missingness. However, before considering missing data mechanisms, two important points are relevant. First, there is no single definition of a missing value. Even if restricting focus to dropout (withdrawal), several possibilities exist. For example, values may be missing as the result of a patient being lost to follow-up, with nothing known about treatment or measurements past the point of dropout. Alternatively, a patient may withdraw from the initially randomized study medication and be given an alternative (rescue) treatment, but with no further measurements taken. Or, follow-up measurements may continue after initiation of the rescue treatment. All these and other scenarios may happen within a single trial, with differing implications for appropriate handling of the data (Mallinckrodt and Kenward, 2009).

Moreover, the consequences of missing values are situation dependent. For example, in a clinical trial for diabetes, if a patient is lost to follow-up halfway through the trial, information needed to understand how well the drug worked for that patient is indeed missing. On the other hand, in a trial for a treatment to prevent breast cancer, if a patient dies from breast cancer midway through the trial, follow-up data are again incomplete; however, information about how well the treatment worked for that patient is not missing because it is known that the treatment did not work.

Knowing that missingness (dropout) may or may not be associated with changes in treatment raises the second important point: how the handling of treatment changes influences outcomes and inferences to be drawn from them. This is, of course, an issue in its own right, but it is also relevant when considering appropriate analyses for incomplete data, especially in the Intention to Treat (ITT) framework that is often the primary basis on which results of confirmatory trials are judged (Mallinckrodt and Kenward, 2009).

While ITT and its alternatives have a direct bearing on the formulation of analyses with missing data, ITT is not a method for handling missing data. Rather, ITT defines the data to be analyzed, and to some extent the inferences drawn from them (Mallinckrodt and Kenward, 2009). An ITT analysis is one in which each patient is assigned for analysis to the treatment group to which he or she was randomized, irrespective of actual subsequent behavior or compliance, and which includes all randomized patients. This definition is the same regardless of whether data are missing or not. The problem, which is discussed in Chapter 3, is how to conform to ITT when some data are missing (Mallinckrodt and Kenward, 2009).

2.2 Missing Data Taxonomy

In order to understand the potential impact of missing data and to choose an appropriate analytic approach for a particular situation, the process (i.e., mechanisms) leading to the missingness must be considered. The following taxonomy of missing data mechanisms is now well established in the statistical literature (Little and Rubin, 2002).

Data are *missing completely at random* (MCAR) if, conditional upon the independent variables in the analysis, the probability of missingness does not depend on either the observed or unobserved outcomes of the variable being analyzed (dependent variable).

Data are *missing at random* (MAR) if, conditional upon the independent variables in the analysis and the observed outcomes of the dependent variable, the probability of missingness does not depend on the unobserved outcomes of the dependent variable.

Data are *missing not at random* (MNAR) if, conditional upon the independent variables in the analysis model and the observed outcomes of the dependent variable, the probability of missingness *does* depend on the unobserved outcomes of the variable being analyzed. Another way to think about MNAR is that if, conditioning on observed outcomes, the statistical behavior (means, variances, etc.) of the unobserved data is equal to the behavior had the data been observed, then the missingness is MAR; if not, then it is MNAR.

With MCAR, the outcome variable is not related to the probability of dropout. In MAR, the observed values of the outcome variable are related to the probability of dropout, but the unobserved outcomes are not. In MNAR, the unobserved outcomes are related to the probability of dropout. The practical implications of the distinction between MAR and MNAR is best appreciated by example. Consider a clinical trial where a patient had meaningful improvement during the first three weeks of the six-week study. Subsequent to the Week-3 assessment, the patient had a marked worsening and dropped out. If the patient was lost to follow-up and there was no Week-4 observation to reflect the worsened condition, the missingness was MNAR. If the Week-4 observation was obtained before the patient dropped out, it is possible the missingness was MAR (when conditioning on previous outcomes).

Mallinckrodt et al. (2008) summarized several key points that arise from the precise definitions of the aforementioned missingness mechanisms. First, given that the definitions are all conditional on the model, characterization of the missingness mechanism does not rest on the data alone; it involves both the data and the model used to analyze them. Consequently, missingness that might be MNAR given one model could be MAR or MCAR given another. In addition, because the relationship between the dependent variable and missingness is a key factor in the missingness mechanism, the mechanism may vary from one outcome to the next within the same data set.

Moreover, when dropout rates differ by treatment group, it would be incorrect to conclude that the missingness mechanism was MNAR and that analyses assuming MCAR or MAR were invalid. If dropout depended only on treatment, and treatment was included in the model, the mechanism giving rise to the dropout was MCAR.

However, given that the missingness mechanism can vary from one outcome to another in the same study, and may depend on the model and method, statements about the missingness mechanism without reference to the model and the variable being analyzed are problematic to interpret. This situational dependence also means that broad statements regarding missingness, and validity of particular analytic methods, across specific disease states are unwarranted.

Moreover, terms such as ignorable missingness can be even more problematic to interpret. For example, in the case of likelihood-based estimation (see Chapter 6), if the parameters defining the measurement process (observed data) are independent of the parameters defining the missingness process (sometimes referred to as the separability or distinctness condition), the missingness is ignorable if it arises from an MCAR or MAR mechanism but is non-ignorable if it arises from an MNAR process (Verbeke and Molenberghs, 2000). In this context, ignorable means the missing-data mechanism can be ignored because unbiased parameter estimates can be obtained from the observed data. However, if other forms of estimation are used, missing data may be ignorable only if arising from an MCAR mechanism. Hence, if missing data are described as ignorable or non-ignorable, this must be done with reference to both the estimation method and the analytic model.

Informative censoring is another term used to describe the attributes of missing data. Censoring is best understood in the context of survival analyses. If the response variable was time to an event, patients not followed long enough for the event to occur have their event times censored at the time of last assessment. Many survival time analyses assume that what caused a patient to be censored is independent of what would cause her/him to have an event. If the outcome is related to the likelihood of censoring, informative censoring is said to have been present. For example, if a patient discontinued because of poor response to treatment, the censoring time was indirectly reflecting a bad clinical outcome.

However, the consequences of informative censoring in regards to longitudinal data analyses are again situation dependent. Informative censoring can arise from MCAR, MAR, or MNAR mechanisms. Therefore, as with describing missingness as ignorable or non-ignorable, additional context must be included in order to appreciate the consequences of informative censoring. And because that context centers on the missingness mechanism, it is most useful to describe missing data via the mechanism (MCAR, MAR, MNAR) rather than the more context-specific terms such as ignorable/non-ignorable or informative/non-informative censoring. Throughout the remainder of this book, missing data are described via the mechanism giving rise to the missingness.

Estimands

3.1 Introduction

An important evolution in the discussions on missing data has been the focus on clarity of objectives. In fact, the first recommendation from the recent National Research Council (NRC, 2010) recommendations on the prevention and treatment of missing data was that the objectives be clearly specified.

The need for clarity in objectives is driven by ambiguities arising from the missing data. As noted in Chapter 2, data may be intermittently missing or missing due to dropout. Patients may or may not be given rescue medications. Assessments after withdrawal from the initially randomized study medication or after the addition of rescue medications may or may not be taken. Whether or not – and if so, how – these follow-up data should be used in analyses and inference is critically important.

Conceptually, an estimand is simply what is being estimated. Components of estimands for longitudinal trials may include the parameter (e.g., difference between treatments in mean change), time point or duration of exposure (e.g., at Week 8), outcome measure (e.g., diastolic blood pressure), population (e.g., in patients diagnosed with hypertension), and inclusion/exclusion of follow-up data after discontinuation of the originally assigned study medication and/or initiation of rescue medication.

Throughout the development of an intervention, the primary goals of the research evolve and therefore the primary estimand may also evolve. Therefore, one estimand cannot be advocated as universally more relevant than others. Rather, the need is to clarify the strengths and limitations of the estimands in order to choose the best one for various situations.

3.2 Hypotheses

Much of the debate on appropriate estimands centers on whether the focus is on efficacy or effectiveness. Efficacy may be viewed as the effects of the drug if taken as directed; for example, the benefit of the drug expected at the endpoint of the trial, assuming patients stayed on drug. This has also been referred to as a per-protocol estimand. Effectiveness in these same settings may be viewed as the effects of the drug as actually taken. This has also been referred to as an ITT estimand.

Referring to estimands in the efficacy-versus-effectiveness context ignores that many safety parameters need to be analyzed. It does not make sense to test an efficacy estimand for a safety outcome. A more general terminology is to refer to hypotheses about efficacy and effectiveness as the de jure (if taken as directed, per protocol) and de facto (as actually taken, ITT) hypotheses, respectively.

Analyses to assess de jure and de facto estimands are presented in Chapter 11. For conceptual understanding here, consider a study to test an intervention in major depressive disorder (MDD). The NRC guidance (NRC, 2010) lists the following five estimands for the MDD and similar settings:

1. *Difference in outcome improvement at the planned endpoint for all randomized participants.* This estimand compares the mean outcomes for treatment versus control regardless of what treatment participants actually received. Follow-up data (after withdrawal of initially randomized medication and/or initiation of rescue medication) are included in the analysis. An example of such a trial was the focal point of a recent editorial on how to address missing data (Fleming, 2011).

Estimand 1 tests de facto hypotheses regarding the effectiveness of treatment policies. However, the most relevant research questions are often in regards to the causal effects of the investigational drugs, not treatment policies, especially early in the research of a drug and in its initial regulatory review. As O'Neill and Temple (2012) noted, including follow-up data as part of the primary estimand is more customary in outcomes trials, whereas in symptomatic treatment trials follow-up data are usually not included in the primary estimand, for the previously noted reasons.

In the ITT framework where inference is drawn based on the originally assigned treatment, including follow-up data when rescue medications are allowed can mask or exaggerate both the efficacy and safety effects of the initially assigned treatments, thereby invalidating causal inferences for the originally assigned medication (Mallinckrodt and Kenward, 2009).

2. *Difference in outcome improvement in tolerators.* This estimand compares the mean outcomes for treatment versus control in the subset of the population who initially tolerated the treatment. This randomized withdrawal design has also been used to evaluate long term or maintenance of acute efficacy. An open label run-in phase is used to identify patients that meet criteria to continue. Those patients that continue are randomized (usually double-blind) to either continue on the investigational drug or switch to control. Including only patients that initially tolerate the drug should reduce dropouts, thereby providing a better opportunity to assess de jure (efficacy) hypotheses. However, estimand 2 focuses on a patient subset and would not be applicable when inference to all patients was desired. Relevance of this estimand is further complicated because in most situations it is not known who will tolerate, and thus all patients must be exposed to the safety risks of the drug, whereas efficacy inferences apply only to the tolerators.

3. *Difference in outcome improvement if all patients adhered.* This estimand addresses the expected change if all patients remained in the study. Estimand 3 addresses de jure hypotheses about the causal effects of the initially randomized drug if taken as directed – an efficacy estimand. Although knowing what happens if a drug is taken as directed is important, it is also hypothetical because there will always be some patients who do not adhere (NRC, 2010).

4. *Difference in areas under the outcome curve during adherence to treatment.*

5. *Difference in outcome improvement during adherence to treatment.*

Table 3.1. *Proposed Estimands and Their Key Attributes*

Estimand	Hypothesis	Inference	Population	Endpoint	Use of Data After Withdrawal of Randomized Study Medication
1	de facto (effectiveness)	Treatment policy	All patients	Planned endpoint	Included in primary analysis
2	de jure (efficacy)	Initially randomized medication	Tolerators	Planned endpoint	Not included in primary analysis
3	de jure (efficacy)	Initially randomized medication	All patients	Planned endpoint	Not included in primary analysis
4	de facto (effectiveness)	Initially randomized medication	All patients	Undefined	Not included in primary analysis
5	de facto (effectiveness)	Initially randomized medication	All patients	Undefined	Not included in primary analysis

Estimands 4 and 5 assess de facto hypotheses regarding the initially randomized drug. These estimands are based on all patients and simultaneously quantify treatment effects on the outcome measure and the duration of adherence. As such, there is no missing data attributable to dropout. However, assessing a drug for effectiveness only during adherence ignores the fact that if patients cannot continue to take the drug they will in many instances have no lasting benefit from it (Permutt and Piniero, 2009; Kim, 2011). In such situations, estimands 4 and 5 overestimate the effectiveness of the drug at the planned endpoint of the trial.

Key attributes of the five estimands are summarized in Table 3.1. Notice that none of the estimands proposed in the NRC guidance (NRC, 2010) address de facto (effectiveness) hypotheses for the initially randomized medication at the planned endpoint of the trial. Therefore, a sixth estimand has been proposed (Mallinckrodt et al., 2012) that may be particularly relevant in the early evaluations and initial regulatory approvals of new medications.

Table 3.2. *An Additional Estimand and Its Key Attributes*

Estimand	Hypothesis	Inference	Population	Endpoint	Use of Data After Withdrawal of Randomized Study Medication
6	de facto (effectiveness)	Initially randomized medication	All patients	Planned endpoint	Likely imputed

6. *Difference in outcome improvement in all randomized patients at the planned endpoint of the trial attributable to the initially randomized medication.* The key attributes of estimand 6 are summarized in Table 3.2, as was done for the other estimands in Table 3.1. Estimand 6 is assessing effectiveness at the planned endpoint, focusing on the causal effects attributable to the initially randomized medications. Conceptually, estimand 1 and estimand 6 require follow-up data. Unlike estimand 1, estimand 6 should be free of the confounding effects of rescue medications. However, ethical considerations often mandate that rescue medications be allowed after patients discontinue randomized study medication.

Conceptually, estimands 3 and 6 both focus on causal effects of the initially randomized medications, in all randomized patients, at the planned endpoint of the trial. However, estimand 3 focuses on what would have happened if patients adhered to treatment and estimand 6 focuses on what was actually observed. Estimand 3 addresses de jure (efficacy) hypotheses and estimand 6 addresses de facto (effectiveness) hypotheses.

3.3 Considerations

Given the confounding effects of rescue medications and the ethical need to allow them, one approach to testing de facto hypotheses is to impute the data after discontinuation of the initially randomized study medication under the assumption that initially randomized active medications have no effect (or a diminished effect) after they are discontinued. This has most commonly been done by imputing values using baseline observation carried forward (BOCF). However, as detailed in Chapter 8, BOCF entails assumptions that are unlikely to hold and it underestimates the uncertainty of imputation. Alternative means to test de facto hypotheses have come into the literature recently and these alternatives are described in Chapter 10.

Another approach to testing de facto hypotheses is to eliminate missing data by making explicit use of dropout in defining a single endpoint outcome that has several components. For example, treatment differences in response rates can be compared where response is considered successful if symptom severity (efficacy) has improved compared with baseline by a certain absolute or relative amount, and if the patient completed the planned assessment interval. All patients who discontinue early are considered treatment failures.

However, Fleming (2011) warned against changing primary endpoints to reduce missing data if it meaningfully compromises the endpoint's clinical relevance. That work used a time-to-event example in which combining a primary outcome with time to discontinuation was not appropriate.

If it is unreasonable to assume that doctors and patients make the same decisions regarding continuation of therapy in a double-blind trial (in which they are unsure about whether the patient is taking drug or placebo) as they would make in actual practice, when the drug and its properties are well known, then dropout may not be appropriate to include as part of a composite outcome (Mallinckrodt et al., 2008).

Part II

PREVENTING MISSING DATA

In contrast to comparing analyses, means to lower dropout are not amenable to study via simulation. Moreover, comparisons from actual clinical trials are of limited use because studies are not done specifically to assess how trial design and conduct influence retention, and thus many confounding factors can mask or exaggerate differences attributable to trial methods. And unlike analytic approaches where multiple methods can be applied to the same data, a study can for the most part be conducted only one way. Comparing design A with design B must therefore be based on between-study comparisons.

Despite these limitations, a number of options can be considered for reducing dropout. These options are discussed in this part of the book, with Chapter 4 focusing on trial design and Chapter 5 covering trial conduct.

Trial Design Considerations

4.1 Introduction

One of the key recommendations from the NRC guidance on prevention and treatment of missing data (NRC, 2010) is that investigators, sponsors, and regulators should design clinical trials consistent with the goal of maximizing the number of participants maintained on the protocol-specified interventions until the outcome data are collected.

However, minimizing missing data is easier said than done. The usefulness of data from actual clinical trials in assessing how design features influence retention is limited because studies are not done with this objective in mind. Therefore, most assessments are on a between-study basis, and thus many confounding factors can mask or exaggerate differences attributable to trial methods. Mindful of these limitations, the NRC Guidance provides a number of suggestions on ways to minimize missing data via trial design, which are discussed in this chapter.

4.2 Design Options to Reduce Missing Data

Run-in Periods and Enrichment Designs

Treatments typically do not work equally well in all patients. If there is a systematic trend for some groups of patients to have better outcomes, this knowledge can be used to reduce dropout by testing the treatment in the subpopulation with the greatest drug benefit. Pretesting and/or selecting patients with greater potential drug benefit prior to randomization is termed enrichment (NRC, 2010).

Run-in designs are similar to enrichment designs. Run-in designs also have an initial period in which a subset of patients is selected. The key difference between run-in and enrichment designs is that response to the experimental treatment is not used to identify the subset in a run-in design (NRC, 2010). Rather, selection is based on compliance, magnitude of placebo response, and so on.

The NRC Guidance notes that although run-ins and enrichment designs may reduce missing data, this benefit typically comes with the trade-off that inferences apply to the subset randomized because responses in the subset will likely be more favorable than in the population as a whole. That is, enrichment and run-ins will likely result in overestimation of benefit and underestimation of harm if inference is drawn on the larger population. Therefore, enrichment designs and run-ins are useful when inference can be restricted to the population subset of patients meeting randomization criteria.

For additional information on and descriptions of run-in periods and enrichment designs, see Fedorov and Liu (2007) and Temple (2005).

Randomized Withdrawal Studies

A randomized withdrawal design is a specific form of enrichment. All patients are initially treated with the experimental medicine or intervention. Only those who remained on the intervention and had a successful outcome are randomized to either stay on the intervention or switch to a control, often placebo. Randomized withdrawal studies typically have longer run-in phases as the goal is to identify patients that sustain an adequate efficacy response. If loss of efficacy after withdrawal constitutes evidence of drug efficacy, a randomized withdrawal trial can generate long-term efficacy data and may have lower rates of dropout. Again, previous experience with relevant situations can guide decisions on the utility of this approach.

Choice of Target Population

Choosing an optimum target population can reduce dropout by ensuring patients are more likely to benefit from the intervention. This is similar to enrichment and run-in designs except the target population is identified based on preexisting knowledge, not based on outcomes from the initial phases of the trial.

The NRC guidance (NRC, 2010) notes that patients doing well on their current treatments may not be good candidates for clinical trial participation as they may be more likely to drop out because of lack of efficacy. Therefore, a good design approach is to include participants who have a minimum baseline level of severity or an unfavorable prognosis if untreated.

Although this principle seems self-evident, the difficulties may lie more in applying the principle than in knowing it. Specifically, even if a useful target population is defined, it may not be easy to ensure that the study sample truly reflects this population. For example, in situations where patient status is determined by evaluators at investigative sites, the site-based raters are typically aware of the study details, previous ratings on patients, and so forth and may be susceptible to expectation bias. Moreover, given the pressure on sites to enroll patients according to aggressive timelines, there may also be (conscious or unconscious) inflation of baseline severity or other inclusion/exclusion criteria so that patients meet entry criteria (Landin et al., 2000).

In many areas of medicine and clinical trials, centralized assessment is standard practice (laboratory analyses, ECGs, toxicological findings, etc). Centralized raters and patient ratings have been proposed as means to improve the quality of psychiatric ratings. Use of highly trained centralized raters via video conferencing is feasible and can improve inter-rater reliability (Shen et al., 2008). The independent perspective on symptom severity or other disease aspects from centralized ratings may also help ensure the target population is indeed enrolled in the trial.

Titration and Flexible Dosing

Protocols that allow flexible dosing to accommodate individual differences in drug response may allow more participants to continue on the assigned treatment by reducing the frequency of dropout because of adverse events or inadequate efficacy (NRC, 2010).

With dose titration, patients initially take a drug at a dose lower than the target or optimal dose in order to reduce adverse events and improve initial tolerability, which can reduce dropout. Titration dosing is often done in clinical practice; hence this design feature may also match real world conditions. However, titration dosing does not allow straightforward assessment of associations between dose and safety or tolerability. Therefore, titration dosing typically is most useful after establishing dose-response relationships.

Flexible dosing may include dose titration, but also allows subsequent dosing adjustments. The basic idea is to set a target dose that patients may titrate to or begin initially. Dose increases above the target dose are allowed for patients with inadequate initial response and decreases below the target dose are allowed if safety or tolerability concerns emerge.

The following example illustrates how flexible dosing may fit into an overall development plan for a drug. Assume phase II studies identified that a particular drug was not effective at 25mg/d in an all-patient cohort, but was effective at both 50mg/d and 100mg/d; 50mg was well tolerated by most patients, but adherence at 100mg/d was less than 50mg/d. Phase III studies could allow patients to begin at 50mg/d, perhaps titrating up from an initial dose of 25mg/d. Only those patients that did not respond adequately to 50mg/d would be increased to 100mg/d. Any patients who had tolerability or safety problems at 50mg/d could have a dose reduction to 25mg/d. Inference would be on the dosing regimen of 25mg/d to 100mg/d, with a 50mg/d target dose.

As with dose titration, flexible dosing may match clinical practice, but inference is on a dosing regimen, not on specific doses. Hence flexible dosing is most applicable to those situations in which inferences on dose-response or specific doses are not required.

Add-on Studies

Add-on studies include designs where in addition to receiving a standard of care patients are randomized to an experimental drug versus control (usually placebo). Add-on designs may reduce dropout attributable to lack of efficacy and in many instances may reflect actual clinical practice (NRC, 2010). However, inference is on the dosing regimen, not on the experimental drug as mono-therapy. In addition, add-on designs generally target a subset of the population with inadequate response to the standard of care because patients doing well on the background treatment are not good candidates to assess the benefits of the experimental drug.

Shorter Assessment Periods

Shorter assessment periods may lead to lower dropout rates compared with longer assessment periods as patients have less opportunity to experience those events that lead to dropout, such as intolerable adverse events. In addition, shorter follow-up reduces the overall burden on patients as the number of clinical visits may be reduced, thereby fostering greater compliance with the planned assessments.

However, shorter treatment periods may not be feasible as longer-term data may be required. Moreover, shorter treatment periods may be less efficient in those instances where the effects of a treatment evolve over time and are therefore larger as the assessment period increases. Use of shorter trials is essentially trading off participants who respond more slowly to study treatment with participants who drop out early. Past experience of similar trials can provide guidance for evaluating this trade-off (NRC, 2010).

The NRC guidance goes on to suggest an alternative wherein primary assessment is based on a shorter assessment period but patients continue in the trial and assessments at subsequent times are taken as secondary.

Rescue Mediations

Use of rescue medications for patients not adequately responding to the initially randomized medications has been strongly encouraged because this can mirror clinical practice and reduce dropout (Fleming, 2011; NRC, 2010). However, as discussed in Chapter 3, the effects of rescue medications can mask or exaggerate the safety and efficacy effects of the originally randomized medications. If this design option is used, the estimand and associated outcome measurements need to be carefully defined in the protocol. For example, time to treatment failure could be the primary outcome and include the use of rescue therapy as an indicator of failure of the initial treatment. This in turn calls for careful specification in the protocol of the circumstances for which rescue therapy is and is not appropriate.

As discussed in Chapter 3, the confounding effect of rescue medication in ITT settings requires that inferences are on the treatment regimen. Therefore, data from patients receiving rescue medications may not be appropriate for drawing causal inference on the initially randomized medications.

Although it has not been discussed at length in the literature, another concern is that readily available rescue medications may reduce *study dropout* but could increase the rate of *medication dropout* – that is, more patients may discontinue the initially randomized medication – which would of course be counter to the primary goal of maximizing the percentage of patients on the initial medications.

Consider the decision to continue randomized medication or not from the point of view of patients in a trial comparing an experimental drug versus placebo. While on randomized medication, the patients know there is a chance they will receive placebo, and if not on placebo then there is a chance that the experimental medication they receive will not be effective. However, if patients opt to discontinue blinded medication, they are sure to receive standard of care.

Therefore, use of rescue medications must be considered carefully. Potential gains from lowering study dropout must be weighed against potential losses from increased medication withdrawal. Most importantly, the use of rescue medications must be considered in light of the primary estimand of the study.

Follow-up Data

Another highlighted recommendation from the NRC guidelines (NRC, 2010), closely linked to use of rescue medications, was collecting follow-up data. Specifically, the panel recommended that "trial sponsors should continue to collect information on key outcomes on participants who discontinue their protocol-specified intervention in the course of the study, except in those cases for which compelling cost-benefit analysis argues otherwise, and this information should be recorded and used in the analysis."

The NRC guidance goes on to state that benefits of collecting follow-up data include assessing the impact of subsequent treatments on outcomes, assessing adverse events after discontinuation of the trial, helping verify assumptions about what outcomes would have been had treatment continued, and of course, if estimand 1 is the primary estimand (see Chapter 3), the follow-up data are part of the primary estimand.

Given the idiosyncratic nature of missing data and its consequences, it is important to consider the specific circumstances of a trial. Certainly, following patients after discontinuation of randomized study medication provides more data, which has value, but is that data worth the cost? Following patients to monitor resolution of adverse effects is clearly necessary for ethical and scientific reasons. However, should patients who discontinue because of adverse effects be given a full assessment battery, or should only safety outcomes be collected? In assessing subsequent treatments, the follow-up data will often be of an observational nature – not arising from randomized comparisons. Therefore, constructing meaningful statistical comparisons may not be straightforward. It is also important to consider exactly how the follow-up data can be used to help verify assumptions about what outcomes would have been had patients stayed on treatment given that the follow-up data arises from patients that did not stay on treatment. Lastly, it is important to recognize that collecting follow-up data does not reduce the amount of missing data for most of the estimands. Therefore, collecting follow-up data should not be seen as a substitute for the most important objective of retaining as many patients as possible on the initially randomized medications.

The point here is not to argue against or for collecting follow-up data. Rather, the intent is to be clear about exactly what collecting follow-up data accomplishes. See Chapter 11 for more illustrations and examples including follow-up data.

Definition of Ascertainable Outcomes

Missing data can arise from the use of outcomes that are undefined for some patients. Therefore, primary outcomes that are ascertainable for all randomized participants should be used. This may require use of composite outcomes (e.g., outcomes that incorporate death as part of the outcome or incorporate use of rescue medication or surgery for initial poor response) (NRC, 2010). However, as noted in Chapter 3, composite outcomes should not be used to avoid the missing data if it compromises the clinical relevance of the outcome.

For composite outcomes that have as one component an ordinal or continuous outcome, other components of the composite, such as study discontinuation or death, might be given the worst outcome rank. In addition, primary outcome measures that require substantial invasive procedures (e.g., liver biopsies) are likely to result in significant missing data, and such outcomes should be avoided whenever possible (NRC, 2010).

Sample Size

The implications of missing data on sample size have been an often overlooked part of the missing data debate. All too often, sample sizes for clinical trials are determined based on simplistic assumptions that do not accurately reflect the impact of missing data. For example, if the anticipated dropout rate is 20%, it is not uncommon for the sample size to be inflated by the same percentage. This approach assumes the missing data arise from a missing completely at random mechanism, which is seldom a justifiable assumption. It also assumes that patients who drop out provide no information about the treatment effect. This assumption would not be true for patients that had some post-baseline assessments included in a repeated measures analysis (NRC, 2010).

The NRC guidance goes on to recommend that the effects of missing data on power cannot be easily assessed analytically, and that simulation studies should be used instead. Power can be evaluated via simulation by generating data using parameters applicable to the particular scenario (time trends, magnitude of treatment effect, rates and timing of missing data, etc.). Data are then analyzed using the relevant primary analysis. The process is repeated, perhaps several thousand times, until reliable estimates of sample size are obtained. It can also be useful to repeat the entire process varying the input parameters across plausible ranges because the input parameters are typically based on estimates and are not known with certainty.

While the aforementioned simulation process has not been routinely done in the past, simulations to assess the operational characteristics of a study are now more common. The NRC guidance concludes by noting that the most worrisome effect of missing values on the inference for clinical trials is bias, and accounting for loss of power from missing data does not address the bias issue.

4.3 Considerations

The consequences of even moderate amounts of missing data are noteworthy and the impact of higher rates of missing data can be profound. Therefore, maximizing the number of participants maintained on the protocol-specified interventions is the most important aspect of mitigating the impact of missing data.

However, objective evidence for the merits of various design approaches to minimize missing data is scarce. Moreover, design options to lower dropout often entail trade-offs. A design feature that reduces the probability of dropout is likely to have consequences in other aspects of the trial. Understanding and managing the trade-offs is key to picking appropriate options for a particular scenario. Given the idiosyncratic nature of missing data and its impacts, it is important to assess the pros and cons of the various options in the specific situation at hand.

Trial Conduct Considerations

5.1 Introduction

The previous chapter on design options to lower rates of missing data noted that evidence to support various approaches was limited because studies are not done specifically to assess how trial design influences retention. Therefore, most assessments are on a between-study basis and thus many confounding factors can mask or exaggerate differences due to trial methods. These same factors limit understanding of how trial conduct influences retention. Again, mindful of these limitations, the recent NRC guidance (NRC 2010) provides a number of suggestions on ways to minimize missing data.

5.2 Trial Conduct Options to Reduce Missing Data

Actions for Design and Management Teams

Trial design should limit participants' burden and inconvenience in data collection. However, once again a trade-off needs to be considered; collecting less data means getting less information. Therefore, study teams need to strike a balance between the conflicting goals of getting the most information possible from a trial and reducing patient burden in order to increase retention (NRC, 2010).

The guidance goes on to list the following options to reduce patient burden: (1) minimize the number of visits and assessments; (2) avoid redundant data collection and collect the minimum amount of information needed to address study objectives; (3) gather data efficiently using user-friendly case report forms and direct data capture (that does not require a clinic visit) whenever feasible; and (4) allow sufficiently large time windows for assessments.

Retention may also be increased by incentives for completing treatment. Providing effective treatments to participants after the trial, or extension phases, or protocols that allow continued access to effective study treatments are options to consider (NRC, 2010).

Site/investigator selection is often based on track records for meeting enrollment guidelines. Selection criteria should be expanded to include rates of complete data while patients are in the trial and in rates of patients that complete the trial (NRC, 2010).

Training provided to sites and patients on the study procedures should emphasize the importance of complete data. And in those instances when follow-up data are collected, the difference between discontinuing data collection should be emphasized (NRC, 2010). An interesting approach to ensure consistent high-quality patient education is to create a short video that is used by every site to educate every patient on key study procedures – and on the importance of complete data.

Investigator payments can be structured to reward completion. The NRC guidance noted that it is acceptable and generally advisable to link a final payment to completion of forms at a study closeout visit. However, the guidance cautioned that it is unethical for patients to complete a study if it exposes them to undue risk. But if there are minimal risks to the participant associated with data collection, it may be acceptable to provide financial incentives to the investigator to continue to collect data, whether or not the participant continues treatment.

Data completeness can be improved by monitoring and reporting it during the course of the trial. The NRC guidance suggested that the information from these assessments be available at investigator meetings and on study Web sites in order to create a climate that encourages study completion. Monitoring can also identify poorly performing sites and the need for remediation or site closure.

A promising tool for preventing patient dropout is the "intent-to-attend" questionnaire (Leon et al., 2007). This short questionnaire asks patients how likely they are to attend their next visit, for example, based on an 11-point (0 – 10) Likert scale. If the patients response is below a pre-chosen threshold, follow-up questions are asked to ascertain what can be done to increase the likelihood of retention. The questionnaire results also provide a potentially useful covariate that can be incorporated into the statistical analyses in order to reduce the potential bias from dropout.

Actions for Investigators and Site Personnel

The NRC guidance also summarized what investigators and site personnel can do to reduce the amount of missing data. Suggestions included emphasizing the importance of completion (and follow-up data, if relevant) during informed consent and informed withdrawal of consent, and providing appropriate incentives for participants. The Code of Federal Regulations requires that study participant compensation is neither coercive nor at the level that would present undue influence (21CFR 50.20). Most IRBs allow cash payments that are slightly backloaded, retaining a small proportion as an incentive for completion.

Patient education should include how their data is important to overall scientific knowledge. This information could be included in a patient video that also covers key study procedures. Participant engagement and retention can be enhanced through newsletters, regularly updated Web sites, study-branded gifts, regular expressions of thanks, and solicitation of input regarding relevant issues of study conduct. Sending visit reminders, as is routinely done in clinical practice, can help avoid missed visits (NRC, 2010).

Clinic visits can be made less burdensome by making the overall experience more pleasant via a welcoming environment, friendly staff that respects the participant's time, provisions for transportation, and availability of on-site diversions for children or provisions for child care.

5.3 Considerations

The NRC guidance recommends that trial protocols establish a minimum rate of completeness for the primary outcome, and monitor progress of the overall trial and individual sites against this benchmark. The guidance included detail on how to choose a suitable benchmark based on past data and what to do if the goal is not met. However, the guidance also noted several factors that make setting appropriate benchmarks difficult. For example, it can be hard to ascertain what procedures a past trial implemented to reduce missing data. Therefore, the dropout rate in a past trial may not accurately reflect expectations for a current trial. Perhaps the main value in having a specific target is that it helps maintain focus on all of the strategies implemented in the trial to help keep rates of missing data as low as possible, regardless of what happened in the past.

Objective evidence on how trial design and trial conduct alternatives influence rates of missing data is scare. Nevertheless, recent literature provides general recommendations that are practical to implement and consistent with good science, even if their impact on missing data rates is not certain. One way to conceptualize an overall approach to preventing missing data is depicted in the following figure. Preventing dropout starts with appropriate choices for study design, study objectives, and primary estimands. With that framework in place, appropriate investigators and patients can be chosen and trained. Trial conduct proceeds mindful of conditions and strategies to maximize retention. And progress is monitored toward study specific goals.

Part III

ANALYTIC CONSIDERATIONS

The merits of statistical analyses can be difficult to understand because there are several important aspects by which to describe the analyses. The common term used to name an analysis often reveals little about these key aspects. For example, it is not uncommon to hear an analysis described simply as last observation carried forward (LOCF). But LOCF is not an analytic method. It is a method for imputing missing values in which the last observed value is used to replace subsequent missing values.

Fully describing a statistical analysis for incomplete longitudinal data requires addressing three key aspects: (1) The method used to estimate the parameters (method); (2) what parameters are to be estimated (model); and (3) choice of data. Choice of data includes whether or not follow-up data are to be included in the analysis and/or by what means, if any, missing values are to be imputed.

This section begins with Chapter 6 that describes general aspects of common methods of estimation used in statistical analyses. While most statisticians will find this review unnecessary, for non-statisticians this material provides the framework necessary to understand different analytic methods, but it is not highly technical. Chapter 7 covers analytic models, with specific emphasis on how to decide what parameters need to be estimated. Chapter 8 outlines the various means of imputing or otherwise dealing with missing values, which is an important part of choosing data.

6

Methods of Estimation

6.1 Introduction

This chapter describes three common methods of statistical estimation: least squares (LS), maximum likelihood (ML), and generalized estimating equations (GEE). In-depth understanding of these methods inherently requires detailed statistical knowledge. However, key concepts can be illustrated using a less technical approach.

The intent is to focus on those key concepts in a nonmathematical manner. Least squares is explained first because it is perhaps the most intuitive method, and then the other methods are explained in relation to least squares. However, prior to discussing these methods, it is useful to consider the frameworks used to draw inference from results.

The three general frameworks for inference are frequentist, Bayesian, and likelihood-based. With frequentist inference, true or false conclusions are drawn from significance tests, or results are expressed in terms of a sample-derived confidence interval. With Bayesian inference, results are expressed in terms of a probability distribution for the parameter being estimated. Likelihood-based inference arises from the assertion that all the information in a sample is contained in probability distributions, called likelihood functions. The extent to which the evidence supports one parameter value or hypothesis against another is therefore equal to the ratio of their likelihoods. From these likelihoods (probabilities) confidence intervals and hypothesis tests can be constructed.

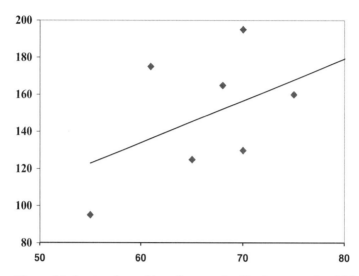

Figure 6.1. Scatter plot and best fit regression line in a scenario with larger errors.

6.2 Least Squares

A standard reference for least squares estimation is Snedecor and Cochran (1989).

It is often reasonable to expect linear relationships between variables. For example, the average weight of humans (y) increases as height (x) increases. However, weight cannot be predicted perfectly from height. For example, body weights can fluctuate as a consequence of experimental error, such as minor fluctuations attributable to time of the last meal or drink prior to weighing, or from equipment that is not calibrated correctly.

A second source of error is that the underlying relationship is not such that there is an exact correspondence between weight and height. For example, people of the same height can be skinny, heavily muscled, or have differing levels of body fat. Even within the same person (adult), weight can fluctuate over time as a result of lifestyle changes, but height remains relatively constant.

Figures 6.1 and 6.2 depict scenarios where the value of y (the variable on the vertical axis) is predicted from x (the variable on the horizontal axis). The line fitted to the data points depicts the average value of y at each x. The slope of the line is called the regression of y on x – that is,

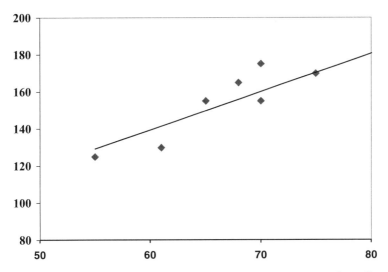

Figure 6.2. Scatter plot and best fit regression line in a scenario with smaller errors.

the average change in y per one unit change in x. Correlation measures the consistency of that relationship and can be visualized as the degree to which the points are scattered around the line. When the points are scattered widely around the line, as in Figure 6.1, the relationship between y and x is less consistent and the correlation is weaker than when the points are clustered closely around the line as in Figure 6.2. However, the average change in y (weight) per unit change in x (height) is approximately the same in the two figures. It is only the degree of consistency that varies.

The degree to which the data points are scattered around the line determines how well the model "fits" the data. The more tightly clustered the points are around the line, the better the fit to the data.

The method of least squares is a procedure that determines the best fit line to the data. Best fit in this case means that the regression line minimizes the distances of the data points around the line. No other line can be drawn that will provide a smaller sum of the distances between the points and the line.

The earlier example is an illustration of simple linear regression, with one dependent variable (y) and one independent variable (x). How-ever, the method of least squares has extensive generalizations and is

Table 6.1. *Calculating Variance and Standard Deviation*

Observation	Mean	Actual Deviation	Absolute Value Deviation	Squared Deviation
120	130	−10	10	100
125	130	−5	5	25
130	130	0	0	0
135	130	5	5	25
140	130	10	10	100
Sum		0	30	250
Variance	=	250 / 5 =	50	
Standard deviation	=	sqrt 50 ~	7	
Average absolute deviation	=	30 / 5 =	6	

not limited to merely finding the best fit line to describe the relationship between two variables. Best fit can be determined for any finite linear combination of specified functions, such as when using several independent variables.

For example, let y be the dependent variable diastolic blood pressure. A model can be fit with multiple independent variables (x). The x variables could include age, gender, ethnicity, and treatment status (drug or control). To further illustrate the concepts of variability and model fit, consider the following two sequences of data:

110	120	130	140	150
120	125	130	135	140

Both have the same mean of 130; however, the first sequence has greater variation about the mean. This leads to the concept of variance, which is a useful tool to quantify how much a set of data fluctuates about its mean. The variance is calculated as the sum of the squared deviations from the mean divided by the number of observations. The standard deviation is the square root of the variance.

Table 6.1 provides an illustration of how variance and standard deviation are calculated for the second, more consistent set of data. It is natural to wonder why *squared* deviations are used to calculate variance – and then take the square root of variance to get the standard deviation. The actual deviations always sum to zero as large positive deviations cancel out large negative deviations. Therefore, actual deviations, despite their intuitive appeal, cannot be used to assess variability. To avoid the cancelling of positive and negative deviations, absolute values can be used. However, the absolute value function is not differentiable, and is not a good function analytically. In contrast, the standard deviation, while not intuitive as a measure of variation, facilitates use of the tools from calculus, which in turn facilitates calculation of probabilities (including p values), construction of confidence intervals, and so forth.

Specifically, the variance equals 50 and the standard deviation is about 7. The standard deviation is fairly close in value to the more intuitive average absolute deviation. However, standard deviation is preferred because it can be associated with probabilities of the normal distribution and average absolute deviations cannot. For example, approximately 2/3 of a population will have values within one standard deviation of the mean and 95% will have values within two standard deviations of the mean. No similar statements can be made regarding average absolute deviations. Again, these probability statements are essential because they form the underpinnings for how such things as p values and confidence intervals are derived.

The method of least squares is intuitive in that it minimizes the squared deviations of predicted values from the actually observed values. That is, the best fit model is the one with the smallest error variance. Least squares has been used broadly across many fields of research because it is a flexible method that can be applied to simple data structures using simple models, or can be adapted to complex situations with complex models.

Data structure and its impact on choice of analytic model are discussed in Chapter 7. A key aspect of data structure is how many observations are taken per experimental unit (subject). A simple data structure would be such as those discussed earlier where there is one observation on the outcome variable per subject. More complex data structures arise when the outcome variable is measured repeatedly on each subject (or experimental unit). Least squares can be adapted to these more complex data structures.

The method of least squares can be subdivided into two categories. Ordinary least squares is what has been discussed thus far and is applicable to simple data structures. Generalized least squares builds on ordinary least squares via some minor algebraic manipulations to accommodate repeated measures on the same subjects over time and the correlations between them.

6.3 Maximum Likelihood

A standard reference for maximum likelihood–based estimation is Harville (1977).

To illustrate maximum likelihood estimation, consider a clinical trial to investigate a new therapy. The primary objective is to determine if the new therapy is effective. For simplicity of illustration, assume that it is not possible to blind the experimental therapy. Hence, the goal is to estimate the proportion of patients that respond to the experimental therapy and compare that percentage to historical data, which suggests that the expected response rate for an ineffective therapy is 20% and the expected response rate for an effective therapy is 60%.

Assume that the trial collects a random sample of m patients, and let y be the number of patients that respond to treatment. The possible values of y are the m+1 integer values 0, 1, 2,... m. Using the principle of maximum likelihood, an estimate of the true population response rate can be obtained and that estimate can be used to decide if the evidence is more consistent with a response rate of 20% that would be expected from an ineffective drug or a response rate of 60% that would be expected from an effective therapy.

Details are illustrated using a convenient, albeit unrealistically small, sample of m=5. Hence the possible outcomes are 0, 1, 2, 3, 4, and 5. Table 6.2 lists the probabilities of obtaining each of these outcomes given a true population frequency of 0.2 (20%) and 0.6 (60%). Although the precise calculation involves the formula for binomial probabilities, which is beyond the current scope, the principle is easily appreciated from flipping a coin. The true probability of getting a head is 50%, but simply due to chance variation, one will not always get 5 heads from every 10 flips of the coin. Similarly, if the true population response rate

Table 6.2. *Probabilities of Binomial Outcomes with True Proportions of 0.2 and 0.6*

True Proportion	Number of Successes					
	0	1	2	3	4	5
0.2	.328	.409	.205	.051	.007	<.001
0.6	.010	.077	.230	.346	.259	.078

is 20% (60%), any one sample is unlikely to have exactly a 20% (60%) response rate. The binomial probability formula can be used to calculate the probabilities for any number of heads in the 10 coin flips, or how many treatment responses to expect in a sample of 5 patients, given a certain true value.

Returning to the hypothetical trial example, assume y = 2 – that is, 2 of 5 patients responded (40%). If the true proportion was 0.2, the probability of this result would be .205 and if the true proportion was 0.6, the probability of this result would be .230. If y = 4, the corresponding probabilities are .007 and .259. Therefore, if y = 2, it is slightly more likely the true value is 0.6 than 0.2. When y = 4 (more generally 3, 4, or 5), a true value of 0.6 is much more likely than a true value of 0.2.

Ignoring now the need to choose between 0.2 and 0.6, what is the most likely value for the true population proportion? Using well-known and straightforward calculus, it can be shown that the best estimate of the true population proportion is the proportion (y/m) obtained in the sample. That is, the principle of maximum likelihood selects as the estimate of a parameter the value that maximizes the likelihood function. In the hypothetical trial example, the maximum likelihood estimate of the response rate is 2/5 = 40%.

Loosely speaking, a likelihood function is the probability distribution associated with the parameter being estimated. Thus, maximum likelihood selects as the parameter estimate the value that has the greatest probability of being the true value, given the observed data. Least squares minimizes the squared deviations (minimizes error variance), whereas maximum likelihood selects the value most likely to be the true value.

It is important to note that using least squares does not mean the errors will be small, only that no other estimates will yield smaller errors. And maximum likelihood does not guarantee the parameter estimates have a high likelihood of being the true value, only that there is no other value of the parameter that is more likely to be the true value, given the data. Under certain conditions (one of them being a y variable that follows a normal distribution), maximum likelihood and least squares yield the same results.

The preceding example focused on a yes/no (binomial) outcome variable. For a normally distributed variable, the appropriate likelihood function is that of the normal probability distribution. This likelihood function includes parameters for the mean and variance. A key implication is that parameters for the mean and variance need to be estimated. When extending this to repeated measures taken in a longitudinal clinical trial, parameters for mean, variance, and covariance (correlation) need to be estimated. See Section 9.3 for an extended example of likelihood analysis on a dataset.

6.4 Generalized Estimating Equations

A standard reference for generalized estimating equations (GEE) is Liang and Zeger (1986).

Intuitively, GEE allows for correlation between repeated measurements on the same patients without explicitly defining a model for the origin of the dependency. As a consequence, GEE is less sensitive to parametric assumptions than maximum likelihood, and is computationally more efficient. Some connections can be drawn between the origins of GEE and maximum likelihood. However, the technical details of these connections go beyond the present scope.

It is especially useful to consider GEE when interest is in estimating the average response over the population ("population-averaged" effects) rather than in predicting patient-specific responses. In addition, GEE may be useful for longitudinal data if difficulties in obtaining proper estimates of the correlations between the repeated measurements are anticipated. However, the relaxed distributional assumptions and non-reliance on correlation structure comes at the price of generally decreased statistical efficiency. That is, all else being equal, parameter estimates from GEE will have greater standard errors than corresponding maximum likelihood estimates. An illustration of GEE is given in Section 9.5.

6.5 Considerations

Common names for statistical analyses may not describe exactly what the method does. Complete understanding of a statistical analysis requires specification of method, model, and choice of data.

In this chapter the fundamental underpinnings of three common methods of statistical estimation were introduced: least squares, maximum likelihood, and GEE. Least squares estimation supports frequentist inference; GEE extends frequentist inference to hierarchical data. And of course, maximum likelihood estimation supports likelihood-based inferences.

The basis for least squares is choosing parameter estimates that minimize the squared deviations between observed data and the outcomes predicted by the analytic model. Maximum likelihood is based on choosing parameter estimates that have the greatest probability of being the true values, given the observed data. Under certain conditions (normally distributed data), least squares and maximum likelihood lead to the same results. Generalized estimating equations arise from the same basis as maximum likelihood, but differ in that GEE requires fewer assumptions about the distribution of the data. The price paid for these relaxed assumptions is reduced efficiency.

The specific properties of the estimation methods relative to missing data are covered in Chapter 9.

Models and Modeling Considerations

7.1 Introduction

The data from longitudinal clinical trials may be as varied as the trials themselves. Verbeke and Molenberghs (2000) provided a detailed and broad review of longitudinal data analyses and Molenberghs and Kenward (2007) provided a similar review specific to clinical trial data.

Given the variety of scenarios that may be encountered in longitudinal clinical trials, no universally best model or modeling approach exists. This implies that the analysis must be tailored to the situation at hand. To an extent, characteristics of the data are driven by the design of the study, and an appropriate analysis follows logically from the design.

Four important characteristics to consider when specifying analyses for longitudinal clinical trials include: (1) the mechanism(s) giving rise to the missing data; (2) the correlations between repeated measures on each patient; (3) the time trends; and (4) the statistical distribution that best describes the likelihood of various outcomes (e.g., normal distribution, binomial, etc.). Analyses appropriate for different missing data settings are discussed in Chapters 9 through 14, whereas the other data characteristics are discussed later in this chapter. These data characteristics influence what parameters need to be estimated, regardless of what method is used to estimate them.

7.2 Correlation between Repeated Measurements

Although the contrast between treatments at a specific time, such as the endpoint assessment, is often the primary focus of clinical trials, interest also exists in the trends over time. Therefore, trials frequently assess patients repeatedly over time.

Many trials have observations taken on the primary outcome measure at a relatively small number of time points. These measurement times are typically fixed, with narrow intervals. Thus measurements may be taken perhaps once per week, with the Week 1 observation mandated to take place between days 5 and 9, the Week 2 observation between days 12 and 16, and so on.

With multiple measurements on the same patients, modeling the (co)variance between the repeated measurements must be considered. The (co)variance arises from three principal sources:

1) Inter-individual variability (i.e., heterogeneity between individual profiles). This variability may be attributable to inherent, patient-specific factors, such as genotype; additional association may arise from unaccounted-for fixed effects, such as age or gender.
2) Further association may arise as a result of time course error (serial correlation), which exists when observations closer to each other in time are more similar than observations further apart.
3) Measurement errors may contribute to random variability. In the longitudinal setting, it is particularly important to consider the potential for error variance to increase or decrease over time (Mallinckrodt et al., 2003).

The relative importance of the various sources of (co)variance can be useful in guiding modeling choices for specific circumstances. For example, in analyses of objective physical measures such as blood pressure or laboratory values, patient-specific factors may have the greatest contribution to within-patient correlations. In these cases a compound symmetric (or random effects or random coefficients) structure may be appropriate because the correlations are equal (or similar) regardless of degree of adjacency. Fixed effects that are not included in the analysis (e.g., patient age or gender) may also give rise to a compound symmetric error structure. In analyses of subjective ratings, such as the Hamilton Depression Rating Scale (Hamilton, 1960), time course errors that decay with increasing distance in time (such as in an autoregressive structure) may also be important.

In many situations, patient-specific effects and serial correlation can be modeled separately, using a mixed-effects model. Laird and Ware (1982) introduced the general linear mixed-effects model to be any model that satisfies

$$
\begin{aligned}
&Y_i = X_i\beta + Z_i b_i + \varepsilon_i \\
&b_i \sim N(0, D) \\
&\varepsilon_i \sim N\!\left(0, \sum\nolimits_i\right) \\
&b_1 \ldots b_n, \ \varepsilon_1 \ldots \varepsilon_n \ \text{independent}
\end{aligned}
\tag{7.1}
$$

where Y_i is the n_i-dimensional response vector for patient i; β is the p-dimensional vector of fixed effects; b_i is the q-dimensional vector of random (patient-specific) effects; X_i and Z_i are $(n_i \times p)$- and $(n_i \times q)$-dimensional matrices relating the observations to the fixed and random effects, respectively; ε_i is the n_i-dimensional vector of residuals; D is a general $(q \times q)$-dimensional covariance matrix with (i,j) element $d_{ij} = d_{ji}$; and $\sum_i$ is a general $(n_i \times n_i)$-dimensional covariance matrix (usually the same for all i). It follows from this model that, marginally,

$$
\begin{aligned}
&Y_i \sim N(X_i\beta, V) \\
&\text{and} \quad V = Z_i D Z_i' + \sum\nolimits_i
\end{aligned}
$$

In other words, mixed-effects models include fixed and random effects. The overall variability (V in the above equation) can be partitioned into parts attributable to the random effects ($Z_i D Z_i'$) and the errors ($\sum_i$). In contrast, analysis of variance models include only fixed effects (apart from the residuals). In clinical trials, the patient-specific (random) effects are seldom the focus. Rather, the trials are typically designed to assess differences in fixed effects, most notably treatment effects. However, accounting for the random effects is needed in order to properly assess the precision of estimates and to make the most appropriate inferences regarding the fixed effects.

A simple formulation of the general linear mixed model (Equation 7.1) can be implemented in which the random effects are not explicitly modeled, but rather are included as part of the error correlation matrix, leading to what could be described as a multivariate normal model. Modeling the random effects as part of the within-patient error correlation structure is the feature that distinguishes the so-called

MMRM analysis from other implementations of mixed-effects models.

The term MMRM, while perhaps convenient in use, does not fully describe the analysis being implemented, and a more precise definition should be used. The statistical properties of MMRM regarding missing data do not arise from how this method models the random effects, but rather from the method of estimation, namely maximum likelihood. For example, MMRM with least squares estimation or GEE would be valid only if the missing data arose from an MCAR mechanism, whereas when using likelihood-based estimation, the assumption is the less restrictive MAR. Therefore, rather than use the term MMRM, it is more appropriate to refer to the method as direct likelihood, with additional description of the model (such as multivariate normal).

In clinical trials where the focus is primarily on the fixed effects, it may be equally appropriate, and more straightforward, to omit explicit modeling of the patient-specific effects and model them as part of the within-patient errors. In such cases the patient-specific effects and serial correlations combine, with or without changes in error variance over time, to yield what is often an unstructured correlation pattern for the within-patient errors.

7.3 Time Trends

Although the longitudinal pattern of treatment effects is usually of interest, a priori knowledge often suggests that the functional form of the response profiles is difficult to anticipate, and linear time trends may not adequately describe the response profiles. Nonlinear trends may arise from inherent characteristics of the particular disease state and drug under study, and/or from trial design features. For example, if titration dosing is used with initial dosing at a subtherapeutic level to reduce adverse events associated with initial tolerability, there may be a lag period with little or no improvement. Conversely, if a drug has rapid onset of a fully therapeutic effect, the beneficial effects may increase rapidly across early assessments and then level off thereafter. In such cases parsimonious approaches to modeling time trends may lead to

inaccurate results and more general models may be preferred (Mallinckrodt et al., 2003).

7.4 Model Formulation

As previously noted, it may be useful to model the random (i.e., patient-
specific) effects as part of the within-patient error correlation structure
if the random effects themselves are not of interest. Handling random
effects in this manner simplifies the analysis while having no (or very
little) impact on inferences of treatment effects (Mallinckrodt et al.,
2008).

Given the typical data structure of clinical trials with a common
schedule of measurements for all patients, a large number of patients,
and a relatively small number of measurement occasions, analyses can
be implemented using a "full multivariate model," featuring an unstructured modeling of time and correlation (Mallinckrodt et al., 2003).

If the number of patients relative to the number of measurement occasions is not large, more parsimonious approaches that require estimation
of fewer parameters are easily implemented. For example, time trends
could be modeled using linear and quadratic effects, and some structured form of the correlation matrix could be fit to the within-patient
correlations. In contrast to "full multivariate models" with unstructured
modeling of time and correlation, the more parsimonious models can
be described as "multivariate models."

A parsimonious model using a structured form of the time trends
can be more powerful than an unstructured model. However, given that
time trends can be difficult to anticipate, parsimonious models can also
be a poor fit. Therefore, in many scenarios, an unstructured modeling
of time and the treatment-by-time interaction provides an assumption-
free approach with regard to time trends, does not require estimation of
an inordinate number of parameters, and can be depended on to yield a
useful result (Mallinckrodt et al., 2003).

An unstructured modeling of within-patient correlations also
removes assumptions (about the correlation structure) and often provides the best fit to the data. However, overly general correlation

structures can lead to analyses that fail to converge. Although failure to converge often results from improperly preparing the data (e.g., two observations on the same patient at the same time point, or poor choice of options in software), a priori specification of the primary analysis should have flexibility to allow alternative models to be fit if an analysis fails to converge because the prespecified correlation structure was too general (Mallinckrodt et al., 2008).

Several approaches can be taken to ensure convergence. First, every attempt should be made to ensure convergence is obtained from a given correlation structure. For example, convergence can be enhanced by using software features such as inputting starting values for parameter estimates, or the use in the initial round(s) (but not final rounds) of iteration algorithms such as Fisher's scoring rather than the Newton-Raphson algorithm, which is the default algorithm in many software packages. Rescaling the data is also an option. If outcomes and covariates are made to fall in ranges in the order of magnitude of unity, interpretations and conclusions will not be changed; but, avoiding manipulation of large or small numbers from a numerical analysis perspective reduces the risk of ill-conditioned matrices, and ultimately, overflow or underflow (Mallinckrodt et al., 2008).

In addition, the protocol can envision one of several model-fitting approaches. A set of structures can be specified and the structure yielding the best fit as assessed by standard model-fitting criteria is considered the primary analysis. However, if it is not appropriate to build models from the same data used to test hypotheses, a series of structures can be specified in a fixed sequence, and the first correlation structure to yield convergence is considered the primary analysis. For example, unstructured could be specified as the structure for the primary analysis, but if it failed to converge, a series of ever-more parsimonious structures appropriate to the situation at hand could be fit until one converges, which would then be considered the primary analysis.

Although these approaches have always yielded a converged analysis, it is reasonable to wonder what effect the true correlation structure in the data and the method of modeling the correlation structure have on results. One study (Mallinckrodt et al., 2004) assessed the effect of correlation structure and how it was modeled in maximum likelihood analyses on Type I error rates and power, and compared results with LOCF. When the correct correlation structure was fit, maximum likelihood provided better control of Type I error and power than LOCF. Although misfitting the correlation structure in maximum likelihood inflated Type I error and altered power, even egregious misfitting of the structure was less deleterious than using LOCF. In fact, simply using an unstructured model in maximum likelihood yielded superior control of Type I error than LOCF in every scenario tested.

In instances where correctness of the correlation structure is a concern, GEE can be used as the method of estimation, rather than maximum likelihood. Alternatively, standard errors and the associated inferences from maximum likelihood analyses can be based on the so-called sandwich estimator, which does not require correct specification of the correlation structure in order to yield valid inferences (Lu and Mehrotra, 2009).

Therefore, maximum likelihood provides flexibility for modeling the within-patient correlation structure, does so in a manner that can be specified a priori, and assures that analysts following those specifications will independently arrive at exactly the same result.

Another aspect of time trends that must be considered is in relation to the other independent variables included in the analysis. The treatment or treatment-by-time intervention effect is clearly the most important effect in many clinical trials. However, other covariates may also be included in the model, and possible interactions with time should be considered. For example, the effect of baseline observation may be included, as patients' responses may depend on their condition at the start of the trial. It is usually preferable to allow a full interaction of the covariate with time, because if not, a restriction is being imposed that the dependence of response on the baseline measure is the same at all time points. Alternatively, both the baseline and post-baseline measures can be treated as response variables (Liang and Zeger, 2000). For other covariates, such as age and gender, it may be appropriate to not include interaction with time because the effects can be taken as constant; however, such decisions need to be justified a priori (Mallinckrodt et al., 2008).

The following example illustrates one way to specify a priori all the details of a likelihood-based analysis such that independent analysts will arrive at exactly the same results. This particular wording specifies the full multivariate approach, with an unstructured modeling of treatment effects over time and within-patient error correlations.

> Mean changes from baseline will be analyzed using a restricted maximum likelihood (REML)-based repeated measures approach. Analyses will include the fixed, categorical effects of treatment, investigative site, visit, and treatment-by-visit interaction, as well as the continuous, fixed covariates of baseline score and baseline score-by-visit-interaction. An unstructured (co)variance structure will be used to model the within-patient errors. If this analysis fails to converge, the following structures will be tested in order as listed: (insert a list of structures appropriate for the specific application ordered from most parameters to fewest). The first correlation structure to yield convergence will be considered the primary analysis. The Kenward-Roger approximation will be used to estimate denominator degrees of freedom and adjust standard errors. Significance tests will be based on least-squares means using a two-sided $\alpha = 0.05$ (two-sided 95% confidence intervals). Analyses will be implemented using (insert software package). The primary treatment comparisons will be the contrast between treatments at the endpoint Visit.

Note that the primary analysis could be based on contrasts at time points other than endpoint, or could be based on the treatment main effects.

7.5 Modeling Philosophies

Collins, Schafer, and Kam (2001) describe restrictive and inclusive modeling philosophies. Restrictive models typically include only the design factors of the experiment, and perhaps one or a few covariates. Inclusive models include, in addition to the design factors, auxiliary variables whose purpose is to improve the performance of the missing data procedure.

Recalling the specific definition of MAR provides rationale for inclusive modeling. Data are MAR if, conditional upon the variables in the model, missingness does not depend on the unobserved outcomes of the variable being analyzed. Therefore, if additional variables are added to the model that explains missingness, MAR can be valid, whereas if the additional variables are not included, the missing data would be MNAR. Little and Yao (1996), Liu and Gould (2002), and Lipkovich, Duan, and Ahmed (2005) provided implementations of inclusive models.

8

Methods of Dealing with Missing Data

8.1 Introduction

Until recently, guidelines for the analysis of clinical trial data provided only limited advice on how to handle missing data, and analytic approaches tended to be simple and ad hoc. The calculations required to estimate parameters from a balanced data set with the same number of patients in each treatment group at each assessment time are far easier than the calculations required when the numbers are not balanced, as is the case when patients drop out. Hence, the motivation behind early methods of dealing with missing data may have been as much to restore balance and foster computational feasibility in an era of limited computing power as to counteract the potential bias from the missing values.

However, with advances in statistical theory and in computing power that facilitates implementation of the theory, more principled approaches can now be easily implemented. This chapter begins with sections describing the simpler methods, including complete case analyses and single imputation methods such as last and baseline observation carried forward. Subsequent sections cover more principled methods, including multiple imputation, inverse probability weighting, and modeling approaches such as direct likelihood.

8.2 Complete Case Analysis

Complete case analyses include only those patients for which all measurements were recorded. This method is simple to describe and because no missing data exist for the patients included in the analysis standard statistical software and simple statistical analyses that are appropriate for complete data can be used.

Unfortunately, the method suffers from severe drawbacks. The loss of information is usually substantial and appreciable bias can result when the missingness mechanism is not MCAR. A simple check of the MCAR assumption is as follows (Little and Rubin, 2002). At each time point, divide the observations into two groups: (1) patients observed at a subsequent assessment and (2) patients missing all subsequent assessments. If data are MCAR, then both groups are random samples from the same population. Failure to reject equality of the distributional parameters (mean and variance) of the samples increases the evidence for MCAR but does not prove it. If the groups are not equal, then MCAR does not hold.

8.3 Simple Forms of Imputation

An alternative way to obtain a data set on which complete data methods can be used is based on filling in (imputing) the missing data rather than deleting the incomplete records. Commonly, the observed values are used in some manner to impute values for the missing observations.

Several strategies may be employed to use observed data as the basis for imputation. Information from the same patient can be used (e.g., last or baseline observation carried forward). Information can be borrowed from other patients – for example, mean imputation where missing values are replaced by the mean value from a corresponding group of patients (e.g., same treatment, same time point). Finally, both within- and between-patient information can be used – for example, hot deck imputation where missing values are imputed from a randomly selected similar record. The term "hot deck" dates back to the storage of data on punch cards and indicates that the information donors come from the same data set as the recipients. The stack of cards was "hot" because it was currently being processed. A standard reference is Little and Rubin (2002).

The user of simple imputation strategies faces several dangers. The imputation model could be wrong, resulting in biased estimates. And even with a correct imputation model, the uncertainty resulting from missingness is often masked by single imputation, leading to an appearance of greater certainty about the result than is actually warranted. In addition, most simple methods require the assumption of MCAR, and some methods require additional and often unrealistically strong assumptions (Verbeke and Molenberghs, 2000).

Widespread use of simple methods for dealing with missing data set a historical precedent that fostered their continued acceptance even as advancements in statistical theory and implementation might have otherwise relegated these methods to the museum of statistics. This was particularly true for the most commonly used approaches in the highly regulated pharmaceutical industry: last observation carried forward (LOCF) and baseline observation carried forward (BOCF).

Continued acceptance of LOCF and BOCF despite strong evidence of their shortcomings was also fostered by the belief that these methods led to conservative estimates of treatment effects. Conservative in this context means not favoring the treatment – that is, underestimating the advantage of treatment over control. Hence, even though it became well known that imputing missing data via LOCF or BOCF yielded biased estimates of treatment effects, that bias was considered appropriate for confirmatory clinical trials of medical interventions because the bias was thought to provide protection against erroneous approval of ineffective interventions.

However, research showed that the direction of bias in LOCF (and BOCF) could not be ascertained from information available at the start of a trial (Molenberghs et al., 2004). Furthermore, a large volume of empirical research showed that the bias from LOCF and BOCF could favor the treatment group and inflate the rate of false positive results, while some of the newer analytic methods were either not biased in these settings or the magnitude of the bias was generally much smaller. (See Mallinckrodt et al., 2008 for a summary of comparisons between LOCF and newer analytic methods in regards to bias from missing data).

Mallinckrodt et al. (2008) used the following to illustrate the difficulties in finding a conservative analytic approach. Consider a method that in truth underestimates the superiority of the superior treatment – that is, underestimates the difference between treatment and control, as LOCF was once perceived to do. Such a method would be conservative when testing a superiority hypothesis of drug versus control for an efficacy outcome. However, a method that underestimates the superiority of the superior treatment necessarily underestimates the inferiority of the inferior treatment. Thus, underestimating treatment effects would be anticonservative in non-inferiority testing and in a superiority test wherein the test agent was inferior to the control. For safety outcomes, underestimating the magnitude of a treatment effect is certainly not conservative.

Hence, it is not surprising that the National Research Council's Expert Panel on missing data, which was convened at the request of the FDA, concluded that LOCF and BOCF were generally not acceptable means of handling missing data (NRC, 2010). However, LOCF and BOCF were still seen as sometimes appropriate methods in the recently issued missing data guidance from the European regulatory body (CHMP, 2010). That guidance suggested that in certain situations LOCF and BOCF can be counted on to yield conservative estimates. Perhaps this is the case for interventions that work by well-known and often studied mechanisms. However, for innovative interventions that work in new ways, the magnitude and direction of bias from LOCF and BOCF would again be unpredictable.

Another motivation for the use of LOCF and BOCF was their intuitive appeal as measures of effectiveness – that is, as a composite of efficacy, safety, and tolerability, rather than as a measure of efficacy (Mallinckrodt et al., 2008). Until now, LOCF and BOCF have been discussed in the context of estimand 3 (Chapter 3) – that is, to test an efficacy hypothesis. Estimands 4 and 5 are formulated based on an alternative interpretation of LOCF, change to last observation, or area under the curve from baseline to last observation.

However, use of these simple imputation methods was also criticized, as, for example, in the following summary from a pharmaceutical industry group consensus paper on choice of the primary analysis (Mallinckrodt et al., 2008). The authors noted that the rate and timing of dropout, which influence the magnitude of treatment estimates obtained via LOCF and BOCF, do not necessarily reflect the true benefit and risk of the drug. While LOCF can in some situations yield attenuated profiles for mean treatment effects when patients drop out, the reduction is not necessarily proportional to the safety risk.

For example, Patient A dropped out late in a trial because of a life-threatening adverse reaction; Patient B dropped out early from a transitory adverse reaction. The impact on estimates of mean change from an LOCF analysis attributable to Patient A's dropout would be small because the last observation was close to the trial's endpoint, allowing considerable time for the benefits of the drug to be realized. The impact from Patient B's dropout would be severe because (in many disease states) little improvement results from a short duration of treatment.

As an even more extreme, but common, example, these same authors considered degenerative conditions such as Alzheimer's disease where the goal is to slow the progression of the illness. Using the last or baseline observation from a patient who dropped out early from the treatment because of an adverse event would actually reward the drug for the adverse event as the patient would appear to have had no further deterioration in condition.

8.4 Multiple Imputation

Multiple imputation was introduced in 1978 (Rubin, 1978) and has become an important approach for dealing with missing data. A standard reference for multiple imputation is Little and Rubin (2002). Applications for multiple imputation initially arose from the field of sample surveys and have spread steadily and now include many applications in clinical trials (Molenberghs and Kenward, 2007).

The key idea behind multiple imputation is to replace each missing value with a set of M plausible values. Each value is a Bayesian draw from the conditional distribution of the missing observation given the observed data, made in such a way that the uncertainty of the imputations is properly taken into account.

The imputations produce M "completed" data sets, each of which is analyzed using a method that would have been appropriate had the data been complete. The model for the latter analysis is called the substantive (or analysis) model, whereas the model used to produce the imputations is called the imputation model (Molenberghs and Kenward, 2007).

Although multiple imputation is most straightforward to use under the assumption of MAR, and most software implementations make this assumption, MI can be applied in MNAR settings. These MNAR applications are particularly convenient when certain classes of pattern-mixture model are used to construct the imputation model. Two examples are Little and Yau (1996) and Thijs et al. (2002). More details on these MNAR approaches are given in Chapter 10.

Molenberghs and Kenward describe the tasks involved in multiple imputation as follows:

1. The missing values are filled in M times to generate M complete data sets.
2. The M complete data sets are analyzed by using standard procedures.
3. The results from the M analyses are combined into a single inference.

The MI estimate is the simple average of the estimates from the M datasets. The precision of the estimates is obtained using Rubin's variance formula (Rubin 1987). This formula involves an intuitive and straightforward combination of within- and between-imputation variability, making the uncertainty of the imputations explicitly evaluable.

Rubin (1987, p. 114) shows that the efficiency of an estimate based on M imputations is such that in many applications as few as five sets of imputations can be almost as efficient as an infinite number of imputations. However, in some applications, such as the clinical trial examples considered by Carpenter and Kenward (2007), substantially more imputations were needed to stabilize the results. Increasing the number of imputations also improves the precision of certain aspects of the imputations (Molenberghs and Kenward, 2007). Given the computational ease in most scenarios, and given that no harm can come from a larger number of imputations, in practice a larger but practical number of imputations, such as 50 or 100, is probably more appropriate than 5.

A number of approaches exist for generating the actual imputations. Details of these approaches are important for statisticians to consider in specific applications, but go beyond our present scope. Additional details can be found in Molenberghs and Kenward (2007, chapter 9). See Section 9.4 for an illustration of multiple imputation on a hypothetical data set. Setting aside these technical ideas for now, consider the following conceptual issues.

One of the strengths of multiple imputation is that the analysis model and the imputation model need not be the same. Meng (1994) introduced the term "uncongenial" for an imputation model that is not consistent with the substantive (analysis) model. There may be variables predictive of missingness that could be included in the imputation model that should not be included in the analysis model because they could confound estimates of the treatment effect. The rationale for inclusive models with additional variables predictive of missingness was described in Section 7.5. The basic idea is that by including the additional variables missingness that would otherwise have been MNAR becomes MAR while retaining the original analysis model that would have been used had the data been complete.

Molenberghs and Kenward (2007) motivate the use of inclusive modeling via an example where a measure of noncompliance was strongly associated with dropout and patients who dropped out were more likely to be non-compliers. The plausibility of MAR would be enhanced by including compliance in the imputation. However, compliance is a post-randomization outcome, and should not be included in the analysis model because it is confounded with treatment.

The importance of assessing sensitivity to underlying assumptions in analyses is stressed in Chapter 12, especially the assumption of MAR. As will be illustrated in subsequent chapters, MI is a convenient method for implementing sensitivity analyses. The same primary likelihood analysis can be kept for the substantive (analysis) model, but the imputation model can be modified to allow for imputations based on MNAR. The approach is flexible and many alternative forms of MNAR models can be considered in the MI framework.

8.5 Inverse Probability Weighting

Inverse probability weighting (IPW) is introduced in this section via an intuitive example patterned after Molenberghs and Kenward (2007), which illustrates how IPW can correct the bias associated with missing data that are not MCAR.

Consider a binary (0/1, failure/success) outcome. Suppose the goal is to estimate the proportion of 1s (successes) in a population represented by a random sample of 12 subjects. Suppose further that all 1s are observed, but only half the patients with 0s are observed, as illustrated below.

Subject	1	2	3	4	5	6	7	8	9	10	11	12
Actual outcome	1	0	0	0	1	0	1	0	0	0	1	0
Observed Outcome	1	?	?	0	1	?	1	0	0	0	1	?

An unbiased estimator of the true population proportion is the observed proportion of successes – if all outcomes are observed, in this case $4/12 = 33\%$. In the example, the proportion of 1s (successes) in the observed data (completers) is $4/8 = 50\%$. Given an MAR or MNAR mechanism, the proportion of 1s observed in the sample is a biased estimate of the true population proportion, and the bias remains no matter how large the sample.

In this hypothetical setting it is known that half of the 0s are unobserved and all the 1s are observed. To compensate, double weight can be given to each 0, leading to the IPW estimate for the probability of a 1 outcome =

$$4/[4 + (2 * 4)] = 4/12 = 1/3;$$

that is, the number of 1s divided by the number of 1s + 2 times the number of 0s, which in this case equals the probability from the complete data.

In practice, the probability of outcomes being missing is not known and must be estimated from the data, using, for example, logistic regression. Therefore, the equality of the estimate and the value that would have been observed if no data were missing will only happen – on average. That is, if the experiment were repeated many times, the average estimate from IPW would equal the estimate from the complete data, but not every estimate would equal the estimate from complete data.

The approach illustrated above is the essence of the approach developed by Horvitz and Thompson (1952), although a number of statistical details have been suppressed for ease of illustration. The method of IPW is most obviously applicable under MAR because there is a direct route to obtaining the probability estimates. The weighting of each observation by the inverse of its corresponding probability of being missing creates in essence a pseudo sample, an estimate of the sample that would have been observed if data were complete.

8.6 Modeling Approaches

Single and multiple imputation approaches, along with IPW, try to "fix" the incomplete data in some way to create the data that would have been observed if no data were missing. Two common alternative approaches are to account for the missingness by jointly modeling the outcome variable of interest and the missingness process (non-ignorable), or to construct an analysis such that the missing data can be ignored (ignorable).

Ignorable Methods

If the missingness arises from an MCAR mechanism, a completers analysis (see Chapter 9) and other methods yield unbiased estimates – that is, the missing data can be ignored. However, because MCAR is not a realistic assumption in most clinical trials, an analysis that can ignore the missingness under the less restrictive assumption of MAR is needed.

Although the specific details may be cumbersome for non-statisticians, the following explanation illustrates how an analysis based on maximum likelihood estimation can ignore the missingness if it arises from either an MCAR of MAR mechanism and yields unbiased results. The explanation is based on factorization of the likelihood function for the joint distribution of the outcome variable and the indicator variable for whether or not a data point is observed. Factorization in this context means that the hypothetical "full" data are split into two parts: the actually observed part and the missing part, which are often described as the measurement process and the missingness process, respectively (Verbeke and Molenberghs, 2000).

For the less mathematically inclined, a more intuitive explanation may be useful. If data are MAR – that is, the observed data explain why values are missing (why patients dropped out) – a likelihood-based analysis yields unbiased estimates and valid inferences from the available data, and the missing data can be ignored. With other methods of estimation, such as GEE and least squares, for the missingness to be ignorable it must arise from an MCAR mechanism. Therefore, the plausibility of assuming the missing data can be ignored is much greater with likelihood-based analyses than with the other methods of estimation.

For those more mathematically inclined, consider the joint distribution of the ith patient's outcomes, denoted Y_i, and the vector of missingness indicators, R_i, to indicate whether or not the outcome is observed or missing; θ and Ψ are parameter vectors describing the measurement and missingness processes, respectively, X_i, W_i, are design matrices associating the respective parameters with the observations. The likelihood function for the full data (to the left of the $=$ sign) can be factored as the marginal distribution of the outcome variable (first term right of $=$ sign) and the conditional distribution of R_i given Y_i, (last term) as illustrated below (Verbeke and Molenberghs, 2000).

$$f(Y_i, R_i|X_i, W_i, \theta, \Psi) = f(Y_i|X_i, \theta)f(R_i|Y_i, W_i, \Psi) \qquad (8.1)$$

Rubin (1976) and Little and Rubin (2002) showed that under MAR and mild regularity conditions (parameters in the measurement and missingness process are functionally independent), likelihood-based (and Bayesian) inferences are valid when the missing data mechanism is ignored. The practical implication is that with likelihood estimation, the correct likelihood can be manipulated from the incompletely observed patients, thereby providing valid parameter estimates and inferences while ignoring the missing data (Molenberghs and Kenward, 2007).

Non-Ignorable Methods

Although missingness in least squares or GEE analyses is ignorable only if the mechanism is MCAR, if least squares or GEE is coupled with a valid form of imputation or weighting, the missingness is ignorable if the mechanism is either MCAR or MAR, which is also the case with likelihood-based estimation. Therefore, non-ignorable methods focus on scenarios where the missingness arises from an MNAR mechanism.

Recall the two ways to think about MNAR are: (1) an association exists between the unobserved outcomes and the probability that those outcomes are missing; and (2) the statistical behavior (means, variances, etc.) of the unobserved data is not equal to the behavior had the data been observed. The obvious but fundamental problem is that the data are missing, so the association between the unobserved outcomes and the probabilities that those observations are missing cannot be evaluated. Nor can the statistical behavior of the data that has not been observed be assessed – only assumption can be made. Conclusions from MNAR analyses are therefore conditional on the appropriateness of the assumed model (Verbeke and Molenberghs, 2000).

Whereas dependence on assumptions is not unique to MNAR analyses, a unique feature with MNAR analyses is that (some of) the assumptions are not testable (Laird, 1994) because the data about which the assumptions are made are missing (Rubin, 1994). See Chapter 10 for a detailed discussion of common MNAR methods, their assumptions, and the consequences these assumptions have for the analyses. See Chapter 12 for details of how MNAR methods can be used in a sensitivity analysis framework.

8.7 Considerations

Simple methods such as complete case analyses, or simple methods of imputation, such as LOCF and BOCF, entail strong and restrictive assumptions that are unlikely to hold in practice. Therefore, these methods are generally not suitable for the primary analysis in clinical trials (NRC, 2010; Mallinckrodt et al., 2008).

Likelihood-based analyses of the available cases (observed data), multiple imputation, and inverse probability weighting are valid under the less restrictive assumption of MAR. Although MAR is often a reasonable assumption in clinical trials, the possibility of MNAR data cannot be ruled out (Molenberghs and Kenward, 2007). However, MNAR methods entail assumptions that cannot be verified from the data.

Part IV

ANALYSES AND THE ANALYTIC ROAD MAP

In the previous section it was noted that describing an analysis requires specifying the method of estimation (Chapter 6), the model (Chapter 7), and choice of data (Chapter 8). In this section, methods, models, and choice of data are combined to illustrate some of the commonly used analyses for incomplete longitudinal clinical trial data (Chapter 9). Chapter 10 covers MNAR methods in greater detail. Chapter 11 focuses on choice of estimand. Chapter 12 discusses how to create an overarching analysis plan that includes sensitivity analyses. Chapter 13 covers analysis of categorical data. Chapter 14 applies these previously discussed topics to the analysis of an actual clinical trial data set. Chapter 15 provides some concluding remarks.

Analyses of Incomplete Data

9.1 Introduction

Describing an analysis requires specifying the method of estimation, the model (which parameters are to be estimated), and choice of data. Choice of data in this context refers to whether or not follow-up data are included, whether or not missing data are imputed, and whether or not observed data are weighted by the inverse probability of being missing.

In this chapter, methods, models, and choice of data are combined to illustrate some of the commonly used analyses for incomplete longitudinal clinical trial data. These analyses are illustrated using small, hypothetical data sets that allow insight into how the methods work when applied to incomplete data. Two data sets are used. The first is a data set with no missing values. The second data set is identical to the first, with the exception that 30% of the endpoint data are missing.

The complete data are listed in Table 9.1. Data are intended to mimic antidepressant clinical trials where symptom severity is based on the Hamilton Depression Rating Scale (Hamilton, 1960). Baseline values are the actual symptom severity scores. Values at times 1, 2, and 3 are changes from baseline, with negative values indicating improvement. Values underlined and in bold are values that were deleted to create the incomplete data set.

In the placebo group, 40% of the endpoint (Time 3) values are missing compared with 20% in the drug group. In the placebo group, the probability of a value being missing is greater for poorer outcomes. In the drug group, one missing value is from a patient that had not improved and the other is from a patient that had robust improvement. The mean

Table 9.1. *Hypothetical Data Set Used to Illustrate Common Analyses for Incomplete Data*

Subject	Treatment	Baseline Value	Changes from Baseline		
			Time 1	Time 2	Time 3
1	Placebo	19	−5	−5	−7
2	Placebo	17	0	3	<u>5</u>
3	Placebo	25	−8	−10	−11
4	Placebo	19	−2	−6	−9
5	Placebo	20	−8	−7	−8
6	Placebo	23	−3	−7	−10
7	Placebo	26	−4	−5	−13
8	Placebo	19	2	**0**	<u>−5</u>
9	Placebo	17	13	**11**	<u>6</u>
10	Placebo	21	−3	−2	<u>3</u>
11	Drug	20	−9	−11	−13
12	Drug	17	1	0	<u>3</u>
13	Drug	21	−3	−4	−10
14	Drug	14	−5	−9	−12
15	Drug	26	−5	−7	−15
16	Drug	18	1	−2	−3
17	Drug	21	−8	−14	<u>**−18**</u>
18	Drug	20	−3	−9	−10
19	Drug	16	−9	−10	−16
20	Drug	23	−6	−8	−11

Note: Underlined values in bold are included in analyses of complete data but are deleted for analyses of incomplete data.

baseline values are 20.6 for the placebo group and 19.5 for the drug group.

Subsequent sections illustrate how common analyses work and how missing data affects their results. However, some basic points regarding longitudinal modeling are illustrated to fix general principles before assessing the specific impact of missing data.

Consider the results in Table 9.2 from likelihood-based analyses of the complete data set. Two models were used. The "simple" model included only treatment, time, and the treatment-by-time interaction. The "base" model included those same effects plus baseline and baseline-by-time interaction.

Table 9.2. *Results from Analyses of Complete Data with and Without Baseline as a Covariate*

Treatment	Time	Simple Model		Model Including Baseline	
		LSMEAN	SE	LSMEAN	SE
0	1	−1.80	1.58	−1.50	1.51
0	2	−2.80	1.67	−2.46	1.57
0	3	−4.90	2.09	−4.39	1.86
1	1	−4.60	1.58	−4.89	1.51
1	2	−7.40	1.67	−7.73	1.57
1	3	−10.50	2.09	−11.01	1.86
Treatment Difference		5.60	2.96 (p = .076)	6.62	2.66 (p = .024)

In the simple model, because the data were completely balanced (same number of observations for each treatment by time combination), the LSMEANS for the treatment-by-time interaction effects are equal to their corresponding raw means. In the model with baseline and baseline-by-time interaction, the LSMEANS do not equal the raw means, thereby reflecting the influence of correcting for differences in baseline values.

The relationship between baseline and change was such that for each one point increase in baseline score, change increased on average approximately one point. Therefore, correcting for the approximately one point higher mean baseline in the placebo group (by including baseline as a covariate) increased the difference between treatments in change at Visit 3 by about one point.

Therefore, the treatment difference was significant in the model that included the covariates (p = .024), but was not significant in the simple model (p = .076).

To further clarify how including baseline as a covariate influenced results, consider the observed and predicted values for selected subjects summarized in Table 9.3. In the simple model, each subject's predicted value equals the corresponding LSMEAN for the treatment-by-time combination. That is, the model contained only group effects; no information unique to individual subjects was in the model. Therefore, individuals' predictions were entirely derived from the group means.

Table 9.3. *Predicted Values for Selected Subjects from Analyses of Complete Data with a Simple Model and a Model that Included Baseline Values as a Covariate*

Subject id	Model	Baseline	Actual Change	Predicted Change
13	Simple	21	−10	−10.50
13	Base	21	−10	−11.92
14	Simple	14	−12	−10.50
14	Base	14	−12	−4.79
15	Simple	26	−15	−10.50
15	Base	26	−15	−17.02

Including baseline as a covariate introduced information specific to individual subjects and the predicted values for each subject were based on a combination of group means and individual patient data (baseline values). The mean baseline value was approximately 20. Subject 13 had a baseline value of 21, close to the overall mean; therefore, the predicted values from the two models were fairly similar for subject 13. However, the baseline value for subject 14 was 14, approximately 6 points lower than the overall baseline mean. The baseline for subject 15 was 26, about 6 points greater than the overall baseline mean. Lower baseline values were predictive of smaller improvements and higher baseline values were predictive of greater improvements. Therefore, when including baseline as a covariate, thereby correcting for baseline differences, the predicted improvement for subject 14 was smaller and the predicted improvement for subject 15 was larger than from the simple model.

9.2 Simple Methods for Incomplete Data

Simple methods of dealing with missing data were discussed in Sections 8.2 (complete cases) and 8.3 (simple forms of imputation). Although such methods are seldom sufficient for realistic scenarios, it is still useful to illustrate them in order to contrast results with more principled methods.

Results from a least squares analyses of completers, LOCF, and BOCF are summarized in Table 9.4. In each analysis, a single observation per subject was included and parameters were estimated using least squares, with a model that included baseline as a covariate and treatment. Results

Table 9.4. *Results from Least Squares Analysis of Incomplete Data Based on Complete Cases, Last Observation Carried Forward, and Baseline Observation Carried Forward*

Analysis	Treatment	LSMEANS	Standard Error	p value
Completers	Placebo	−9.28	1.40	
	Drug	−11.54	1.20	
	Difference	2.26		.260
LOCF	Placebo	−3.65	1.87	
	Drug	−10.95	1.87	
	Difference	7.3		.014
BOCF	Placebo	−5.45	1.66	
	Drug	−9.35	1.66	
	Difference	3.90		.118
Complete data	Placebo	−4.39	1.86	
	Drug	−11.01	1.86	
	Difference	6.62		.024

from the complete data (no missing values) are included at the bottom of the table for reference.

In the completers and BOCF analyses, the difference between treatments was smaller, and in LOCF the treatment differences was larger, than the difference in the complete data. Standard errors from the completers analysis were also smaller than in the complete data, as the smaller sample size was more than offset by reduced variability.

To further clarify how missing data are handled in these simple analyses, refer back to the data in Table 9.1 and consider the data used by the various methods for subjects 8 and 10. In the complete data, Subject 8 had a two-point worsening at Time 1 followed by a return to the baseline level at Time 2, and a five-point improvement at Time 3. However, in the incomplete data, Time 2 and Time 3 were missing. In the complete data, Subject 10 had small improvements at Time 1 and Time 2, but worsened at Time 3. In the incomplete data, the Time 3 observation was missing.

In the completers analysis, all data from subjects 8 and 10 were excluded. Because subjects doing poorly were more likely to drop out, and there was more dropout in the placebo group, the within-group changes from the completers analysis was greater than in the complete data, and the differences between treatments was smaller than in complete data.

With both LOCF and BOCF, the imputed value for subject 8 was less favorable and the imputed value for subject 10 was more favorable than the corresponding value from the complete data. The within-group changes from both LOCF and BOCF were less than from the complete data; however, the difference between groups was greater for LOCF and smaller for BOCF compared with the complete data.

9.3 Likelihood-Based Analyses of Incomplete Data

Likelihood-based estimation was introduced in Chapter 6. The basis for ignoring missing data in a likelihood-based analysis, so long as it is either MCAR or MAR, was explained in Chapter 8. Some general principles of modeling complete data were illustrated in Section 9.1. This section further illustrates specifically how a likelihood-based analysis accounts for missing data.

Consider first hypothetical Subject 1 in Group 1. Assume the visitwise means for Group 1 reflect consistent, gradual improvement. Assume Subject 1 was doing poorly and dropped out. Simple means based on the observed data in Group 1 after the time Subject 1 dropped out will be biased because the poor data from Subject 1 is not present at later visits. In a repeated measures likelihood-based analysis, the means for Group 1 at the visits after Subject 1 dropped out are adjusted to reflect that had the subject stayed in the trial her observations would likely have continued to be worse than the group average. But the analysis predicts that this subject would have had some additional improvement because subjects in Group 1 tended to improve over time.

Next consider hypothetical Subject 2, also from Group 1, who was doing better than average prior to dropout. In a likelihood analysis, subsequent means are estimated to reflect that had Subject 2 stayed in the trial his improvement would likely have continued to be greater than the average for that group. The group means are adjusted to reflect the anticipated performance of the subjects that dropped out. The magnitudes of these "adjustments" are determined mathematically from the data. Additional details can be found elsewhere (Cnaan et al., 1997; Verbeke and Molenberghs, 2000; Molenberghs and Kenward, 2007).

The following example, using the hypothetical data in Table 9.1, illustrates the handling of incomplete longitudinal data via a maximum

Table 9.5. *Results from Likelihood-Based Analyses of Complete and Incomplete Data, with a Model Including Baseline as a Covariate*

Treatment	Time	Complete Data		Incomplete Data	
		LSMEANS	SE	LSMEANS	SE
0	1	−1.50	1.51	−1.65	1.50
0	2	−2.46	1.57	−2.23	1.74
0	3	−4.39	1.86	−5.71	1.81
1	1	−4.89	1.51	−5.03	1.52
1	2	−7.73	1.57	−7.93	1.71
1	3	−11.00	1.86	−11.71	1.65
Endpoint Treatment Difference		6.62	2.66 (p = .024)	6.00	2.48 (p = .044)

likelihood analysis. The analysis model included treatment, time, and the treatment-by-time interaction as categorical effects, with baseline value and baseline-by-time interaction included as covariates. With incomplete data, information from the observed outcomes is used via the correlation between the repeated measurements to provide information about the unobserved outcomes, but missing data are not explicitly imputed. Results are summarized in Table 9.5.

In the complete data, the difference between treatments at the endpoint visit was 6.62, and the corresponding standard errors and p values were 2.66 and .024, respectively. In the data set with missing values, the difference between treatments at the endpoint visit was 6.00 and the corresponding standard errors and p values were 2.48 and .044, respectively. Mean changes in both groups were slightly greater from analyses of the incomplete data than from the complete data. All else being equal, the standard error for the endpoint treatment contrast from complete data is expected to be smaller than the standard error from incomplete data because of the smaller number of observations in the incomplete data. However, in the example data, the variation was less in the incomplete data, and therefore the standard error of the endpoint treatment contrasts was also smaller.

To further clarify how missing data are handled in likelihood-based analyses, consider the observed and predicted values for selected subjects, summarized in Table 9.6. The sequence of observations on Subject 8 in the complete data was 2, 0, and −5; only the first data point was

Table 9.6. *Predicted Values for Selected Subjects from Analyses of Complete Data with a Simple Model and a Model that Included Baseline as a Covariate*

Subject id	Data	Baseline	Actual Change	Predicted Change	Standard Error
8	Incomplete	19		−2.02	3.35
8	Complete	19	−5	−3.26	1.97
10	Incomplete	21		−6.24	3.26
10	Complete	21	3	−5.30	1.86

present in the incomplete data. Therefore, in the incomplete data, the only observation on Subject 8 was a two-point worsening whereas the group average at Time 1 was an improvement of about 1.5 points. Therefore, predicted values for Subject 8 at Time 2 and Time 3 from the incomplete data reflected continued below-average performance with smaller improvements than the corresponding group averages. In the complete data, the Time 2 observation of 0 was again below the group average, but the Time 3 observation of −5 was approximately the group average. Therefore, in the complete data, the predicted improvement for Subject 8 was closer to the group average than in the incomplete data. As expected, the standard error of the predicted value at Time 3 was greater from analyses of the incomplete data than from the complete data.

The sequence of observations on Subject 10 in the complete data was −3, −2, and 3; only the first two observations were present in the incomplete data. Therefore, in the incomplete data, the observations on Subject 10 were similar to the group averages for those time points. Consequently, the predicted value for Subject 10 at Time 3 was close to the group mean, reflecting the anticipation that this subject would have continued to perform at about the group average if the subject had stayed in the trial. In the complete data, the Time 3 value for Subject 10 was a 3-point worsening compared with the group mean of a 5-point improvement. As a consequence of this additional unfavorable outcome, the predicted value for Subject 10 at Time 3 from complete data reflected a somewhat less optimistic outcome than the corresponding change predicted from the incomplete data. As expected, the standard error of the predicted value at Time 3 was greater from analyses of the incomplete data than from the complete data.

The aforementioned examples illustrate restricted models that include (typically) only the design factors of the experiment and a parsimonious set of covariates. It is possible to include auxiliary variables in likelihood-based analyses. This could be done by either adding the variable(s) as a covariate or as a second response variable to create a multivariate analysis.

However, multivariate analyses can become complex and computationally intensive. Moreover, including auxiliary variables that are post-baseline, time-varying covariates – possibly influenced by treatment – can cause confounding with the treatment effect, leading to erroneous inferences. As will be seen in the next section, multiple imputation may be a better framework for making use of auxiliary variables because they can be included in the imputation step to account for missingness but then not included in the analysis step to avoid confounding with the treatment effects (Molenberghs and Kenward, 2007).

9.4 Multiple Imputation-Based Methods

Another approach for incomplete data that also assumes MAR is multiple imputation. Results from multiple imputation (MI) are expected to be similar to results from a likelihood-based analysis when the imputation and analysis model in MI match the model from the likelihood analysis. Specifically, given the similar models, as the number of patients (N) and the number of imputations (M) increases, the results from the two analyses converge, apart from small differences attributable to the asymptotic approximations involved (Molenberghs and Kenward, 2007).

With finite M, the maximum likelihood estimators are more efficient than MI, although the difference may be small. Nevertheless, when using restricted modeling, direct likelihood may be preferred over MI. However, MI may be preferred over direct likelihood when covariates are missing because likelihood analyses ignore the entire record, whereas MI can impute the missing covariate and make use of the record. In addition, MI may be preferred when using inclusive models, for which likelihood analyses may be impracticable or awkward (Molenberghs and Kenward, 2007).

Table 9.7. *Results from Multiple Imputation–Based Analyses of Incomplete Data*

Endpoint Contrast Complete Data			Endpoint Contrast Incomplete Data		
LSMEANS	SE	P Value	LSMEANS	SE	P Value
6.62	2.66	.024	6.15	6.04	.324

The following example, using the hypothetical data in Table 9.1, illustrates the handling of incomplete longitudinal data via multiple imputation. The imputation model included baseline severity and previous responses on the outcome variable, with the number of imputations set at 5 (m = 5). The analysis model was the same as in the likelihood analysis and included treatment, time, and the treatment-by-time interaction as categorical effects, with baseline value and baseline-by-time interaction included as covariates. Key results are summarized in Table 9.7. The previously reported results from the complete data are again included for reference.

In the complete data, the difference between treatments at the endpoint visit was 6.62, and the corresponding standard errors and p values were 2.66 and .024, respectively. In the data set with missing values, the difference between treatments at the endpoint visit when imputing missing values via MI was 6.15, and the corresponding standard errors and p values were 6.04 and .324, respectively. Estimates from the individual data sets ranged from a 15-point advantage for drug to a 2-point advantage for control.

The standard error for the endpoint contrast in the MI analysis of the hypothetical data was more than twice the magnitude of the standard error from direct likelihood. The disparity was particularly dramatic here given only 14 subjects with endpoint data. In most realistic clinical trial scenarios, the disparity in efficiency will be much smaller.

To further clarify how missing data are handled in MI, consider the observed and imputed values for selected subjects that are summarized in Table 9.8.

The sequence of observations on Subject 8 in the complete data was 2, 0, and −5; only the first data point was present in the incomplete data. Therefore, in the incomplete data, the only observation on Subject

Table 9.8. *Observed and Imputed Values for Selected Subjects in Multiple Imputation Analysis of Incomplete Data*

Imputation	Time 1	Time 2[1]	Time 3[2]
1	2	1	−12
2	2	2	−6
3	2	10	11
4	2	4	29
5	2	11	−24
			Mean = −0.4, SD = 20
1	−3	−2	−16
2	−3	−2	−8
3	−3	−2	−5
4	−3	−2	2
5	−3	−2	−14
			Mean = −8.2, SD = 7.2

[1] Time 2 values are imputed for subject 8 and observed for subject 10.
[2] Time 3 values are imputed for both subject 8 and subject 10.

8 was a 2-point worsening whereas the group average at Tine 1 was an improvement of about 1.5 points. Therefore, imputed values for Subject 8 at Time 3 averaged −0.4, which reflected continued below-average performance with smaller improvement than the corresponding group average. In the complete data, the Time 3 observation of −5 was approximately the group average. Therefore, in the complete data, the predicted improvement for Subject 8 was closer to the group average than in the incomplete data.

The sequence of observations on Subject 10 in the complete data was −3, −2, and 3; only the first two observations were present in the incomplete data. Therefore, in the incomplete data, the observations on Subject 10 were similar to the group averages for those time points. The average imputed value for Subject 10 at Time 3 of −8.2 was slightly greater than the group mean of approximately −5. In the complete data, the Time 3 value for Subject 10 was a 3-point worsening. As a consequence of this additional unfavorable outcome, the predicted value for Subject 10 at Time 3 from complete data reflected a somewhat less optimistic outcome than the corresponding change predicted from the incomplete data.

Imputed values for Subject 8 were based on only baseline and Time 1, whereas for Subject 10, imputed values were based on baseline, Time 1, and Time 2. Consequently, the standard deviation of the Time 3 imputed values for Subject 8 was nearly threefold than that for Subject 10.

9.5 Weighted Generalized Estimating Equations

A standard reference for weighted generalized estimating equations (wGEE) is Robins, Rotnitzky, and Zhao (1995). See Section 8.6 for a review of generalized estimating equations.

With fully observed data, parameter estimates from GEE are consistent and asymptotically normal regardless of the assumed within-patient (longitudinal) correlation structure. When data are missing, this property no longer holds and estimates may depend strongly on the assumed correlation structure.

Furthermore, it was previously noted that GEE is valid only under MCAR. However, weighting the observations in GEE by the inverse probability of dropout (i.e., inverse probability weighting, or IPW) can correct for MAR missingness without the need for assumptions about the correlation structure, as is required in a likelihood-based analysis. Instead, all that is required for valid MAR analyses using wGEE is a suitable model for the missingness process (dropout) (Molenberghs and Kenward, 2007).

The relaxed assumptions on correlation structure come at the price of generally decreased efficiency compared with a likelihood-based analysis, because information from completers is the basis for estimation and inference in GEE. The wGEE approach can be an easier-to-implement alternative for marginal models in analyses of categorical variables where direct likelihood (or related methods) is difficult to implement. More details on analyses of categorical outcomes are given in Chapter 13.

The basic approach with wGEE is to estimate the probability of dropout for each patient at each visit, given the patient was observed at the previous visit. The probabilities are then accumulated over visits. Each observation is weighted by the inverse of the probability of dropout and a suitable analysis is conducted.

The probability of dropout can be modeled via logistic regression, such as could be implemented via PROC GENMOD in SAS. It is

Table 9.9. *Results from Weighted GEE Analyses of Incomplete Data*

Endpoint Contrast Complete Data			Endpoint Contrast Incomplete Data		
LSMEANS	SE	P Value	LSMEANS	SE	P Value
6.62	2.66	.024	wGEE	6.75	1.93	.0005
			wGEE (trim)	5.78	1.85	.0018
			GEE	5.34	1.76	.0024

customary to include in the dropout model the outcome variable at the previous occasion or a set of previous occasions, and treatment group. Other covariates predictive of dropout can be included. The inverse probabilities from the logistic regression are used to weight the observations for the analyses of the outcome variable. Analysis of the outcome variable can also be conducted in PROC GENMOD with appropriate link functions, error distributions, and correlation structures.

Although wGEE is valid under MAR whenever the probability model is correctly specified, this analysis may yield estimates with high variance when some weights are large – that is, when the probability of dropout is high. The augmented wGEE approach (see Section 9.6) can be used to partially remedy this weakness. Furthermore, weights can be trimmed or bucketed into strata with weightings based on a strata mean or median.

The following example, using the hypothetical data in Table 9.1, illustrates the handling of incomplete longitudinal data via wGEE. The dropout model included baseline severity, treatment, previous responses on the outcome variable, and the interaction of previous responses with treatment. The analysis model was the same as in the likelihood analysis and included treatment, time, and the treatment-by-time interaction as categorical effects, with baseline value and baseline-by-time interaction included as covariates. Results are summarized in Table 9.9. The previously reported results from the complete data are again included for reference.

The results from the dropout model showed that as improvement increased, probability of dropout decreased. Hence, subjects with unfavorable observations were more likely to drop out. In the complete data, the difference between treatments at the endpoint visit was 6.62, and the corresponding standard errors and p values were 2.66 and .024, respectively. In the corresponding data set with missing values, the wGEE

Table 9.10. *Individual Subject Data and Weighting Factors for Weighted GEE Analyses*

			Changes from Baseline			
Subject	Treatment	Baseline Value	Visit 1	Visit 2	Visit 3	Weight
1	Placebo	19	−5	−5	−7	1.03
2	Placebo	17	0	3	*	2.34
3	Placebo	25	−8	−10	−11	1.00
4	Placebo	19	−2	−6	−9	1.21
5	Placebo	20	−8	−7	−8	1.00
6	Placebo	23	−3	−7	−10	1.09
7	Placebo	26	−4	−5	−13	1.05
8	Placebo	19	2	*	*	1.12
9	Placebo	17	13	*	*	1.00
10	Placebo	21	−3	−2	*	6.06
11	Drug	20	−9	−11	−13	1.20
12	Drug	17	1	0	*	13.3
13	Drug	21	−3	−4	−10	1.27
14	Drug	14	−5	−9	−12	1.19
15	Drug	26	−5	−7	−15	1.27
16	Drug	18	1	−2	−3	1.29
17	Drug	21	−8	−14	*	18.9
18	Drug	20	−3	−9	−10	1.24
19	Drug	16	−9	−10	−16	1.18
20	Drug	23	−6	−8	−11	1.25

Note: The bolded asterisks (*) indicate missing values.

estimate of the difference between treatments at the endpoint visit was 6.75, and the corresponding standard errors and p values were 1.93 and .0005, respectively.

To further clarify how missing data are handled via inverse probability weighting, first consider the results from unweighted GEE and trimmed wGEE analyses in Table 9.9 and the data weighting factors for subjects in Table 9.10.

Most of the subjects that dropped out had weights greater than 2.0. Drug group Subjects 12 and 17 had the largest weights. These subjects had unusual profiles in that they dropped out from a group that had a low probability of dropout. The weight for Subject 17 was greater than for Subject 12 because Subject 17's robust early improvements suggested a lower probability of dropout than for Subject 12 who had no improvement.

In the placebo group, the weights for Subjects 8 and 9 were close to 1 even though they dropped out. Dropout was more common in the placebo group and Subjects 8 and 9 were getting worse, not better. These observations did not receive large weightings because the profiles were not unusual. Subject 10 had a fairly large weight of approximately 6 that resulted from the unusual profile of dropout despite reasonable early improvement.

Returning to the results in Table 9.8, the unweighted analysis yielded a treatment contrast of 5.34, with a standard error of 1.76. Therefore, weighing the observations increased the magnitude of the treatment difference, but also increased the standard error as a consequence of additional uncertainty associated with estimating the weights.

A key assumption of wGEE is a stable weight model. Given the smallness of the data set, even one aberrant weight on an influential observation can influence results. Trimming weights may be useful to curb the effects of unstable weights. To illustrate the principle of trimming, the maximum weight was capped at 7.0. Therefore, the weights on drug group Subjects 12 and 17, which were two and three times greater than the largest placebo subject weight, were trimmed to barely bigger than the largest placebo weight. Not surprisingly, the results from the trimmed analysis were intermediate to the fully weighted and unweighted results.

9.6 Doubly Robust Methods

Common references for the emerging area of doubly robust methods include Carpenter, Kenward, and Vansteelandt (2006) and Tsiatis (2006).

It was previously noted that wGEE is less efficient than likelihood-based methods. The efficiency of wGEE can be improved by augmenting the weighted generalized estimating equations with the predicted distribution of the unobserved data given the observed data (Molenberghs and Kenward, 2007).

The estimators obtained by solving the augmented and weighted GEE are semi-parametric estimators because they do not model the entire distribution. For this reason, semi-parametric estimates are generally not as efficient as maximum likelihood estimators obtained using the correct model, but they remain consistent where maximum likelihood estimators from a misspecified parametric model are inconsistent (Molenberghs and Kenward, 2007).

Augmentation also introduces the property of double robustness. To understand double robustness, recall that efficient IPW estimators require three models:

1. The substantive (analysis) model that relates the outcome to explanatory variables and/or covariates of interest.
2. A model for the probability of observing the data. This is usually a logistic model of some form.
3. A model for the joint distribution of the partially and fully observed data, which is compatible with the substantive model in (1).

If model (1) is wrong – for example, because a key confounder is omitted – then estimates of all parameters will typically be inconsistent.

The intriguing property of augmented wGEE is that if either model (2) or model (3) is wrong, but not both, the estimators in model (1) are still consistent. However, doubly robust methods are fairly new, with few rigorous simulation studies or real data applications in the literature and no standardized software. Given these limitations, and the complexity of doubly robust methods, no further illustrations are provided.

9.7 Considerations

In this chapter common analyses of incomplete data under the assumption of MAR were illustrated using a small, hypothetical data set. In practice, the setting, data characteristics, and analyses may be more complex than the simple setting used here. However, simplicity allowed illustration of key principles and the inner workings of the analyses.

In practical situations, when implemented in a similar fashion, likelihood-based, multiple imputation–based, and weighted GEE analyses tend to yield similar results, with the degree of similarity increasing with size of the data set, and in the case of MI, the number of imputations.

Likelihood-based methods tend to be more efficient. Hence, in situations where restrictive models are to be used, likelihood-based methods may be somewhat preferred. However, when more flexibility is desired for the imputation model in MI or the dropout model in wGEE, such as whenever inclusive modeling is used, MI and wGEE are generally preferred.

MNAR Analyses

10.1 Introduction

Although the assumption of MAR is often reasonable in clinical trials, the possibility of MNAR data is impossible to rule out (Verbeke and Molenberghs, 2000). Therefore, analyses valid under MNAR are needed. Analyses in the MNAR framework try in some manner to model or otherwise take into account the missingness process. However, moving beyond MAR to MNAR poses fundamental problems.

In MAR it is assumed that the statistical behavior of the unobserved data is the same as if it had been observed, such that the unobserved data can be predicted from the observed data. As was noted in Section 8.6, the fundamental difficulty with any MNAR method is that the characteristics and statistical behavior of the missing data are unknown.

The inescapable fact is that moving beyond MAR to MNAR can only be done by making assumptions. Conclusions from MNAR analyses are therefore conditional on the appropriateness of the assumed model. While dependence on assumptions is not unique to MNAR analyses, a unique feature with MNAR analyses is that (some of) the assumptions are not testable (Molenberghs, Kenward, and Lesaffre, 1997) because the data about which the assumptions are made are missing (Laird, 1994). Importantly, the consequences of model misspecification are more severe with MNAR methods than with other (e.g., MAR) methods (Little, 1995; Laird, 1994; Rubin, 1994; Draper, 1995, Kenward, 1998). Hence, no individual MNAR analysis can be considered definitive. Not surprisingly then, many statistical methodologies have been proposed to analyze data in the MNAR setting.

General classes of MNAR methods have arisen from different factorizations of the likelihood functions for the joint distribution of the outcome variable and the indicator variable for whether or not a data point is observed. Factorization in this context means that the hypothetical "full" data are split into two parts: the actually observed part and the missing part, which are often described as the measurement process and the missingness process, respectively.

Review papers that describe in detail, compare, and critique these models include Little (1995), Hogan and Laird (1997), Little and Rubin (2002), Diggle et al. (2002), Fitzmaurice et al. (2004), and Molenberghs and Kenward (2007).

The following sections describe general aspects of selection models, shared parameter models, and pattern mixture models, which are some of the commonly used MNAR methods. Describing these more complex methods is inherently more complex than the descriptions of the MAR analyses in Chapter 9, and some statistical notation is unavoidable. The following terminology is used to describe and compare the methods.

Subject i is to be measured at times $j = 1, \ldots, n$

Y_{ij} is the measurement taken on subject i at time j, where j can take on the values $1 - n$

R_{ij} is an indicator variable taking on the value of 1 if Y_{ij} is observed, 0 otherwise.

Group Y_{ij} into a vector $Y_i = (Yo_i, Ym_i)$

Yo_i contains Y_{ij} for which $R_{ij} = 1$,

Ym_i contains Y_{ij} for which $R_{ij} = 0$.

Group R_{ij} into a vector R_i commensurate with Y_{ij} such that all 1s are paired with the Yo_i and the 0s are paired with the Ym_i

D_i is the time of dropout

Ψ = Parameters describing missingness process

θ = Parameters describing measurement process

10.2 Selection Models

A standard reference for selection models is Diggle and Kenward (1994).

A selection model can be thought of as a multivariate model, where one variable is the continuous efficacy outcome from the primary analysis and the second variable is the binary outcome for dropout modeled via logistic regression. The joint distribution of the ith patient's outcomes (Y_i) and the missingness indicators (R_i) is factored as the marginal distribution of Y_i and the conditional distribution of R_i given Y_i.

$$f(Y_i, R_i|\theta, \psi) = f(Y_i|\theta)f(R_i|Yo_i, Ym_i, \psi) \qquad (10.1)$$

In contrast to ignorable models where it is assumed the missingness process is independent from the measurement process (conditional on the measurements), an MNAR selection model explicitly ties together the measurement and missingness processes as the outcome variable (Y) from the measurement model is a predictor variable in the dropout (missingness) model.

A standard formulation of the selection model is illustrated as outlined in the NRC guidance on the prevention and treatment of missing data (NRC, 2010). Assume the full-response data comprise (Y1, Y2), and the objective is to compare the Y2 means in each group. Further, assume Y2 is missing on some individuals. A parametric selection model might assume that the full-response data follows a bivariate normal distribution and the "selection mechanism" part of the model follows a logistic regression.

Parametric selection models can be fit to observed data, even though there is no empirical information about several of the model parameters. For example, there is no information about the association between the values of R (0 or 1) and Y2 because Y2 is missing in all instances when $R = 0$.

The model can be fit because of the parametric and structural assumptions imposed on the full-data distribution. Therein lays both the benefit and the danger of selection models. The benefit is that the selection model (and other MNAR methods) allows estimation without data, of course, under the assumptions that the model is appropriate. The danger is that the appropriateness of the model and its assumptions cannot be verified from the data.

10.3 Shared Parameter Models

Standard references for shared parameter models include Wu and Carroll (1988) and Wu and Bailey (1989).

In a shared-parameter model, a set of latent variables, latent classes, and/or random effects is assumed to drive both the Y_i (measurement) and D_i (missingness, in this case time to dropout) processes. An important version of this model further asserts that, conditional on the latent variables, Y_i and D_i are independent. A shared-parameter model can be thought of as a multivariate model, where one variable is the continuous efficacy outcome from the primary analysis and the second is (typically) a proportional hazards time to event analysis for dropout.

Specifically, the full data likelihood can be factored similar to a selection model as the product of the marginal outcome distribution $f(Y_i|b_i)$ and the conditional distribution of D_i given Y_i and b_i.

$$f(Y_i, D_i, b_i) = f(Y_i|b_i)f(D_i|Y_i, b_i)f(b_i) = f(Y_i|b_i)f(D_i|b_i)f(b_i) \quad (10.2)$$

The dropout and measurement models are again linked as the same random effects are in both outcome and dropout models. As in selection models, there are again untestable assumptions, namely that, conditional on the latent (that is, unobserved) random effects, Y_i and D_i are independent. This assumption is untestable because Y_i is missing in each instance when D_i is prior to the end of the trial.

10.4 Pattern-Mixture Models

Standard references for pattern mixture models include Little (1993, 1994, 1995).

Pattern-mixture models were originally developed based on the reverse factorization of the full data likelihood as for the selection model. Hence, the full data likelihood is the product of the measurement process conditional on the dropout pattern and the marginal density of the missingness process.

$$f(Y_i, R_i | \theta, \psi) = f(Y_i | R_i, \theta) f(R_i | \psi) \qquad (10.3)$$

The pattern-mixture model fits a response model for each pattern of missing values such that the observed data is a mixture of patterns weighted by their respective probabilities. Results are pooled over the various patterns for final inference. These models can be viewed from an imputation perspective in which missing values Y_m are imputed from their predictive distribution.

Pattern-mixture models in this imputation context are by construction under-identified, that is over-specified. For example, say the goal of a study is to estimate the difference between treatments at endpoint. Three patterns are identified: early dropouts, late dropouts, and completers. Missing values for the endpoint from the early and late dropouts are to be imputed. But in order to do that, information must be borrowed because there is no information about the endpoint visit in the early and late dropout patterns.

This problem can be resolved through the use of identifying restrictions wherein inestimable parameters of the incomplete patterns are set equal to (functions of) the parameters describing the distribution of other patterns. Alternatively, pattern indicators can be used in the regression functions, so as to reach a more parsimonious model. This is especially useful with sparse patterns. Nevertheless, the focus here is on imputation-based approaches.

Although completely arbitrary restrictions can be used by means of any valid density function over the appropriate support, strategies that imply links back to the observed data are likely to have more practical relevance (Molenberghs and Kenward, 2007). Three specific and common identifying restrictions all use data from patients that remained in the study at time t to identify the distribution for those patients that discontinued (NRC, 2010). These restrictions are:

CCMV: Complete Case Missing Values, where information that is unavailable is always borrowed from the completers.

NCMV: Neighboring Case Missing Values, where information that is unavailable is borrowed from the nearest identified pattern.

ACMV: Available Case Missing Values, where information that is unavailable is borrowed from all patterns in which the information is available, weighted according to the proportion of patients in each pattern from which information is borrowed.

ACMV is important in that with this approach the analysis assumes MAR. In addition, a general family of restrictions can be defined as non-future-dependent missing value restrictions (NFD) where one conditional distribution per incomplete pattern is left unidentified. In other words, the distribution of the "current" unobserved measurement, given the previous measurements, is unconstrained. In practice, this can be accomplished by using data only up to and including the time point being imputed as the basis for estimating parameters for the imputation model.

When information is borrowed in the NFD family via CCMV or NCMV, the mechanism is MNAR. Therefore, comparing results from ACMV with NFD-CCMV or NFD-NCMV allows an assessment of sensitivity of results to departures from MAR.

Although not commonly seen thus far in the literature, it is also possible to define patterns by reason for dropout rather than time of dropout; or, as described in Section 10.5, patterns can be defined by treatment group.

10.5 Controlled Imputation Methods

Recently, another family of methods increasingly referred to as controlled imputation has been discussed in the literature and used in practice. Little and Yao (1996), Carpenter and Kenward (2007), Ratitch and O'Kelly (2011), and Teshome et al. (2012) proposed imputation approaches that can be thought of as specific versions of pattern-mixture models. The common idea in each of these approaches is to construct a principled set of imputations that exhibit a certain statistical behavior, typically a departure from MAR, in order to assess either sensitivity of de jure estimands or as a primary means to assess de facto estimands.

In MAR implementations of MI, separate imputation models are used for the drug and control arms (in a two-arm study). For MNAR analyses, one subfamily of approaches within controlled imputation, referred to as reference-based imputation, uses one imputation model developed from data in a reference group (e.g., placebo, or standard of care) and uses that model to impute missing data for both the drug and control arms.

Using one imputation model for both treatment arms will typically diminish the difference between the arms compared with MAR approaches that use separate imputation models for each arm. The intent is to generate a plausibly conservative efficacy estimate that can be used to define the lower bound of values for the set of plausible sensitivity analyses; or, to generate an estimate of effectiveness that reflects a change in or discontinuation of treatment.

In addition to reference-based imputation, imputation can also be controlled by repeated adjustment to provide a progressively more severe stress test to assess how extreme departures from MAR must be to overturn the primary result. For example, the analysis can assume that patients who discontinued had outcomes that were worse than otherwise similar patients that remained in the study (NRC, 2010; Carpenter and Kenward, 2007). The difference (adjustment) in outcomes between dropouts and those who remain can be a shift in mean or slope, and is referred to as delta.

Typically, only the experimental arm is delta-adjusted whereas the control arm is handled using an MAR-based approach. Delta-adjustment can be applied to only the first visit with missing data or to all visits with missing data; delta-adjustment also can be applied as part of a visit-by-visit imputation or after completion of all imputations.

Delta-adjustment after imputation simply subtracts a constant from the imputed values and the adjustment at a visit does not influence imputed values at other visits. With delta-adjustment in visit-by-visit imputation, missing values are imputed as a function of both actually observed and previously imputed delta-adjusted values. In this setting, delta-adjustment influences imputed values at the visit to which it is applied and also influences imputed values at subsequent visits through the imputation model. Delta-adjustment applied to every visit in a visit-by-visit imputation results in an accumulation of adjustments and thus implies a greater departure from MAR than delta-adjustment at a single visit.

Specific details of one approach, placebo multiple imputation (pMI), are included later here, with logical extensions following for other variations. The pMI approach has also been termed copy reference, because information is taken from a reference group, which in this specific case is placebo.

In pMI, multiple imputation is used to replace missing outcomes for drug- and placebo-treated patients who discontinued using multiple draws from the posterior predictive distribution estimated from the placebo arm. Specific details are provided here.

To set up the imputation model, define observed patient-specific covariates (X) and partially observed outcomes (Y_{obs}) whose joint distribution drive the imputation mechanism for missing outcomes. Given T measurement occasions, let $y_i = \{y_{i,obs}, y_{i,mis}\}$, the $1 \times T$ outcome vector containing for the i-th patient k_i observed outcomes and $T - k_i$ unobserved outcomes, and x_i is a $1 \times P$ vector of fully observed covariates.

Given a monotone pattern of missingness, Bayesian regression employing factorization of the multivariate normal density for the data with monotone missingness pattern (Rubin, 1987), such as is available is SAS PROC MI (SAS, 2003), provides an easy way to impute the missing values. The basic idea is to estimate the parameters for the imputation model using only data from the placebo arm and then use those parameters to impute missing values for both the drug-treated and placebo-treated patients. Partially observed outcomes from treated patients are used when imputing their missing outcomes as follows.

Data are processed sequentially by repeatedly calling SAS PROC MI to impute missing outcomes at visits t=1,..,T.

1. *Initialization.* Set $t=0$ (baseline visit)
2. *Iteration.* Set $t=t+1$. Create a data set combining records from placebo and treated patients with columns for covariates X and outcomes at visits 1,..,t with outcomes for all treated patients set to missing at visit t and set to observed or imputed values at visits 1,..,t−1.
3. *Imputation.* Run Bayesian regression in SAS PROC MI on this data to impute missing values for visit *t* using previous outcomes for visits

1 to $t-1$ and baseline covariates. Note that only placebo data will be used to estimate the imputation model because no outcome is available for treated patients at visit t.

4. Replace imputed data for all treated patients at visit t with their observed values, whenever available. If t < T then go to Step 2, otherwise proceed to Step 5.

5. Repeat steps 1–4, m times with different seed values to create m imputed data sets.

6. *Analysis.* For each completed data set, using the model as would have been applied had the data been complete.

The confidence intervals and p values are obtained from the multiple datasets using Rubin's combining rules (Rubin, 1987), as implemented in SAS PROC MI ANALYZE (SAS, 2003).

The following (Table 10.1) is an illustration of pMI using the hypothetical data originally introduced in Chapter 9. The values in parenthesis were missing in the original data and represent imputed values from pMI.

The endpoint treatment contrast estimated via pMI was −5.08, with corresponding standard error and p values of 2.96 and .089, respectively. Recall from Chapter 9 that the maximum likelihood estimate from the complete data was 6.62; from the incomplete data, the maximum likelihood estimate was 6.00, with corresponding estimates from wGEE and standard MI of 6.75 and 6.15, respectively.

Two views may be taken of the quantity estimated by pMI: (1) as an assessment of effectiveness, assuming patients who discontinued before the endpoint received no or reduced pharmacological benefit after dropout (estimand 6; see Chapter 3); and (2) as a worst reasonable case assessment of efficacy – the outcome that would have been observed had the patient stayed on drug.

In the effectiveness context, if a patient had experienced benefit from the drug prior to dropping out, the more favorable observed outcomes from that patient would influence the imputed values in pMI such that imputed outcomes would be more favorable than if observed outcomes were less favorable. However, the carrying forward of this drug benefit is commensurate with the correlation structure implied by the imputation

Table 10.1. *Hypothetical Observed and Imputed Data to Illustrate Placebo Multiple Imputation*

Subject	Treatment	Baseline Value	Visit 1	Visit 2	Visit 3
				Changes from Baseline[1]	
1	Placebo	19	−5	−5	−7
2	Placebo	17	0	3	$(-9, -1, 3, 14, 0)$
3	Placebo	25	−8	−10	−11
4	Placebo	19	−2	−6	−9
5	Placebo	20	−8	−7	−8
6	Placebo	23	−3	−7	−10
7	Placebo	26	−4	−5	−13
8	Placebo	19	2	$(-4, -2, 9, 2, 1)$	$(-11, 0, -4, 4, 0,)$
9	Placebo	17	13	$(9, -2, 8, -5, 8)$	$(12, 7, -4, 6, 8)$
10	Placebo	21	−3	−2	$(-5, -3, 8, -4, -5)$
11	Drug	20	−9	−11	−13
12	Drug	17	1	0	$(-4, -10, 3, 6, -7)$
13	Drug	21	−3	−4	−10
14	Drug	14	−5	−9	−12
15	Drug	26	−5	−7	−15
16	Drug	18	1	−2	−3
17	Drug	21	−8	−14	$(0, -7 -12, 2, -8)$
18	Drug	20	−3	−9	−10
19	Drug	16	−9	−10	−16
20	Drug	23	−6	−8	−11

[1] Values in parentheses were missing from the original hypothetical data and represent values imputed as per placebo multiple imputation.

model, which would typically result in a declining drug benefit after discontinuation.

A declining drug benefit after discontinuation would be appropriate for assessing effectiveness of drugs with fairly long half-lives. However, the flexibility of controlled imputation allows tailoring to specific clinical settings. For example, the imputations can be controlled to have the treatment effect immediately disappear after discontinuation, as might be appropriate for an acute pain medication with a short half-life. Imputations can also be controlled so that changes in drug- and control-group patients are the same after dropout, as might be appropriate for drug with disease modification properties.

In the effectiveness context, pMI is a more principled alternative to LOCF and BOCF. First, pMI properly accounts for uncertainty via use of multiple imputation whereas BOCF and LOCF underestimate uncertainty because they use single imputation. In addition, pMI accounts for study effects and placebo effects because it uses the placebo group for reference whereas BOCF and LOCF assume there are no study effects and no placebo effects because they assume no change after baseline or last observation. Given that in many situations patients either tend to improve or worsen during the course of a trial, depending on whether the treatment goal is to alleviate symptoms or to prevent worsening, the assumptions of no placebo or study effects are unlikely to be valid.

Teshome et al. (2012) compared LOCF, BOCF, and pMI in regards to estimating effectiveness in simulated scenarios where there was no difference between drug and control for patients that dropped out and with varying levels of drug – control differences in completers. The pMI approach had less bias than either LOCF or BOCF in all scenarios examined.

10.6 Considerations

The NRC guidance on prevention and treatment of missing data summarizes the advantages and disadvantages of selection models and pattern mixture models as follows (NRC, 2010).

The selection model framework is intuitive. If MAR is plausible, a likelihood-based selection model leads directly to inference based solely on the model for the full-data response, and inference can proceed via maximum likelihood estimation. However, specifying the relationship between the probability of nonresponse and the outcome of interest, which typically is done on the logit scale, is less intuitive. Moreover, the predictive distribution of missing responses is typically intractable, making it difficult to understand exactly how the missing observations are being treated for a given model. Furthermore, selection models are sensitive to parametric assumptions about the full data distribution. This concern can be alleviated to some degree via semi-parametric selection models. Many of these same comments can be applied to shared-parameter models.

Pattern-mixture models are also intuitive in that it is natural to think of respondents and nonrespondents as having different outcome distributions. Pattern-mixture models are transparent with respect to how missing observations are being imputed because the within-pattern models specify the predictive distribution directly. Pattern-mixture models can present computational difficulties for estimating treatment effects because of the need to average over missing data patterns; this is particularly true of pattern-mixture specifications involving regression models within each pattern.

Controlled imputation methods hold promise as sensitivity analyses for testing efficacy hypotheses and for testing effectiveness hypotheses. These methods, as is generally the case for pattern mixture approaches, involve transparent and easy-to-understand assumptions that are plausible in common clinical trial scenarios. However, these approaches are relatively new and more experience would be useful.

Choosing Primary Estimands and Analyses

11.1 Introduction

Previous chapters focused on estimands, methods of and models for estimation, and means for dealing with missing data. These topics are now considered jointly in order to appreciate the interactions between them. For example, different estimands applied to the same data may yield greater or fewer missing values, which can influence the method of estimation and the validity of assumptions.

In the following section, the six estimands introduced in Chapter 3 are discussed with regard to data choices, methods of estimation, and assumptions. To refocus the discussion, key attributes of the 6 estimands are summarized in Table 11.1.

11.2 Estimands, Estimators, and Choice of Data

Estimand 1

Difference in Outcome Improvement at the Planned Endpoint for all Randomized Subjects

Estimand 1 tests a de facto (effectiveness) hypothesis at the planned endpoint of the trial, based on all randomized patients. Data after discontinuation of the initially randomized study medication and/or initiation of rescue medication are included in the primary analysis. Given the confounding influences of the follow-up data, inferences are based on the treatment regimen, not the initially randomized treatments.

The missing data literature does not rigorously address what to do about missing follow-up data. However, extrapolation from similar

Table 11.1. *Estimands and Their Key Attributes*

Estimand	Hypothesis	Endpoint	Use of data after withdrawal of randomized study medication and/or initiation of rescue medication
1	de facto (effectiveness)	Planned endpoint	Included
2	de jure (efficacy)	Planned endpoint	Not included
3	de jure (efficacy)	Planned endpoint	Not included
4	de facto (effectiveness)	Change to last observation	Not included
5	de facto (effectiveness)	Area under curve baseline-last	Not included
6	de facto (effectiveness)	Planned endpoint	Likely imputed

circumstances suggests that the missing follow-up data could be imputed using the controlled imputation approaches described in Section 10.5, with the reference group being the standard of care/rescue therapy. The usefulness of the imputation model can be assessed by comparing the imputed values to the actually observed follow-up data.

For simplicity, estimation of estimand 1 is illustrated later in this chapter assuming no follow-up data are missing, and data are analyzed via maximum likelihood. Data used for this analysis are listed in Table 11.2. These are the same hypothetical data as in Table 9.1, with the values bolded and underlined being the data that was deleted to create the incomplete data. Values bolded, underlined, and in parenthesis are the hypothetical values representing the influence of rescue medication – that is, the follow-up data.

Results from the maximum likelihood analysis of the data in Table 11.2, using the follow-up data, are summarized in Table 11.3. The analysis used a restrictive model that included treatment, time, and the treatment-by-time interaction as categorical effects, with baseline value and baseline-by-time interaction included as covariates. To facilitate ease of comparison, results from complete and incomplete data originally summarized in Table 9.5 are also included in Table 11.3.

When including follow-up data in the analysis, the difference between treatments and the variability in the data decreased over time compared

Table 11.2. *Hypothetical Data Used to Illustrate Estimation of Estimand 1*

Subject	Treatment	Baseline Value	Changes from Baseline[1]		
			Visit 1	Visit 2	Visit 3
1	Placebo	19	−5	−5	−7
2	Placebo	17	0	3	**5 (−13)**
3	Placebo	25	−8	−10	−11
4	Placebo	19	−2	−6	−9
5	Placebo	20	−8	−7	−8
6	Placebo	23	−3	−7	−10
7	Placebo	26	−4	−5	−13
8	Placebo	19	2	**0 (−5)**	**−5 (−10)**
9	Placebo	17	13	**11 (−4)**	**6 (−9)**
10	Placebo	21	−3	−2	**3 (−12)**
11	Drug	20	−9	−11	−13
12	Drug	17	1	0	**3 (−8)**
13	Drug	21	−3	−4	−10
14	Drug	14	−5	−9	−12
15	Drug	26	−5	−7	−15
16	Drug	18	1	−2	−3
17	Drug	21	−8	−14	**−18 (−12)**
18	Drug	20	−3	−9	−10
19	Drug	16	−9	−10	−16
20	Drug	23	−6	−8	−11

[1] The bolded, underlined values are included in analyses of complete data but are deleted for analyses of incomplete data.

Table 11.3. *Results from Likelihood-Based Analyses of Complete and Incomplete Data*

Treatment	Time	Complete Data LSMEANS (SE)	Incomplete Data LSMEANS (SE)	Follow-up Data Included LSMEANS (SE)
Placebo	1	−1.50 (1.51)	−1.65 (1.50)	−1.50 (1.50)
Placebo	2	−2.46 (1.57)	−2.23 (1.74)	−4.80 (1.12)
Placebo	3	−4.39 (1.86)	−5.71 (1.81)	−10.20 (0.94)
Drug	1	−4.89 (1.51)	−5.03 (1.52)	−4.60 (1.50)
Drug	2	−7.73 (1.57)	−7.93 (1.71)	−7.40 (1.12)
Drug	3	−11.01 (1.86)	−11.71 (1.65)	−11.00 (0.94)
Endpoint Treatment Difference		6.62 (2.66, p = 024)	6.00 (2.48, p = .044)	0.80 (1.33, p = .555)

with results from the incomplete data. The difference between treatment regimens at endpoint was less than 1 point, and was not significant (p = .555). Such results would be expected when poorer-performing subjects are more likely to use rescue therapy and there is a difference between treatments in the percentage of subjects rescued. The rescue therapy generally improves the responses of poorer-performing subjects, thereby reducing the difference between treatments and increasing the similarity (reducing variability) of responses at endpoint.

Estimand 2

Difference in Outcome Improvement in Tolerators

Estimand 2 tests a de jure (efficacy) hypothesis at the planned endpoint of the trial, in those subjects who originally tolerated the drug during a run-in phase. Data after discontinuation of the initially randomized study medication and/or initiation of rescue medication are not included in the primary analysis.

The difference between estimands 2 and 3 is only the choice of data. For estimand 2, a run-in phase is used to identify subjects who tolerate the drug, and it is only the tolerators who are randomized to drug versus control, thereby hopefully reducing the amount of missing data, but also limiting inference to those who tolerate. In contrast, estimand 3 is based on all subjects and uses a standard design, without the run-in phase. Given these similarities, all comments in the next section about estimand 3 can also be applied to estimand 2, mindful of the required design differences.

Estimand 3

Difference in Outcome Improvement if all Subjects that Tolerated or Adhered

Estimand 3 tests a de jure (efficacy) hypothesis at the planned endpoint of the trial, in all randomized patients. Data after discontinuation of the initially randomized study medication and/or initiation of rescue medication are not included in the primary analysis, but could be included, if available, to test secondary objectives. Importantly, the same design could be used to assess estimands 1 and 3, with follow-up data included for estimand 1 but not estimand 3.

The goal for estimand 3 is to estimate what would have been observed had the subjects adhered to the originally assigned treatment. The key missing data assumption is that the missing data arise from an MAR mechanism. If data are MAR, then the observed data can be used to predict the unobserved data.

Estimation of estimand 3 was illustrated in Chapter 9 using maximum likelihood (Section 9.3), multiple imputation (Section 9.4), and weighted GEE (Section 9.5). Results from the maximum likelihood analysis are relisted for convenience in Table 11.3. The difference between treatments increased over time and was statistically significant at endpoint. The standard errors also increased over time, reflecting the reduced sample sizes attributable to subject dropout.

Estimand 4

Difference in Areas under the Outcome Curve During Adherence to Treatment

Estimand 4 tests a de facto (effectiveness) hypothesis in all randomized patients. Similar to estimand 5, this is not a time-specific estimand, such as at the planned endpoint of the trial. Rather, the estimand is based on the sum of changes from baseline to last observation, regardless of when the last observation was obtained. As such, dropout or time to dropout is an inherent part of the estimand, and there are no missing data and therefore no assumptions regarding missing data. Estimand 4 can be obtained from the same data as used for estimand 3.

Given no data are missing, estimation of estimand 4 can proceed using simple methods of estimation, such as least squares, with a simple model that includes, for example, only treatment and baseline. Applying this analysis to the hypothetical data, the means for drug and placebo were 21.87 and 10.62, respectively, with corresponding standard errors of 3.71, yielding a p value for the difference between treatments of .048.

Estimand 5

Difference in Outcome Improvement During Adherence to Treatment

Estimand 5 is similar to estimand 4, except that rather than summing the changes during adherences, only the last observation is used. Estimand 5 tests a de facto (effectiveness) hypothesis in all randomized patients. This is again not a time-specific estimand, such as at the planned endpoint of the trial. Rather, the estimand is based on the last observation, regardless of when it was obtained. As such, dropout or time to dropout is an inherent part of this estimand and there are no missing data and therefore no assumptions regarding missing data are needed.

Estimation of estimand 5 was illustrated in detail in Chapter 9 (Section 9.2) using least squares estimation and a model that included treatment and baseline. In that section, the method was referred to as last observation carried forward (LOCF). While LOCF can also be interpreted in the context of estimand 3, truly carrying observations forward to the planned endpoint, the numerical result for the last observation analysis for estimand 5 is identical; the only difference is in the interpretation of the result.

The difference between treatments in the hypothetical data set was 7.30 (p = .014). Therefore, the treatment effect based on estimand 5 was slightly greater than for estimand 3 based on the maximum likelihood analysis of incomplete data.

Estimand 6

Difference in Outcome Improvement in all Randomized Patients at the Planned Endpoint of the Trial Attributable to the Initially Randomized Medication

Estimand 6 tests a de facto (effectiveness) hypothesis at the planned endpoint of the trial, based on all randomized patients. Data after discontinuation of the initially randomized study medication are included in the primary analysis. However, given that inference is to be drawn on the initially randomized treatments, rescue medications are not allowed. If follow-up data could be obtained without rescue medications, estimation of estimand 6 can proceed as previously described for estimand 1. The only difference between these two estimands is the allowance or restriction of rescue medication.

However, in many circumstances ethical needs mandate the use of rescue medications; therefore, data after discontinuation of the initially randomized medications will often need to be imputed. Estimation of estimand 6 was illustrated in Section 10.5, using the so-called placebo multiple imputation (pMI) approach. Data for both the drug- and placebo-treated subjects are imputed using a model developed from the placebo group only. Therefore, the follow-up data are imputed based on the assumption of either no maintained benefit or diminishing benefit after discontinuation or initiation of rescue medication. The completed data sets resulting from the imputations can be analyzed with any suitable analysis for complete data.

Maximum likelihood estimation was used in conjunction with pMI for the analyses of the hypothetical data in Section 10.5, yielding an endpoint treatment contrast of -5.08, with corresponding standard error and p values of 2.96 and .089, respectively.

11.3 Considerations

Conclusions drawn from a data set are contingent on the estimand. In analyses of the hypothetical data, with estimand 1 the difference between treatment regimens was small and did not approach significance. For estimands 4, 5, and 6, which assessed effectiveness of the originally assigned medication, treatment differences were significant or approached significance. For estimand 3, which assessed efficacy of the originally assigned medication, the difference between treatments was significant.

Each estimand has strengths and limitations; there is no universally best choice. The choice of the primary estimand should be driven by the scientific question. Fleming (2011) warned against choosing primary endpoints simply to reduce missing data if it meaningfully compromises the endpoint's clinical relevance.

For example, the utility of estimand 5 – change to last observation – hinges on the medical relevance of the last observation. For therapies that treat the symptoms of chronic illnesses, the last observation is probably less meaningful than for therapies that can modify or eliminate the disease. The utility of estimand 1 hinges on the relevance of treatment regimens rather than individual treatments.

Stage of development is another potential influence on the choice of estimand. Across the development of a particular intervention there may be a shift in focus requiring a commensurate change in primary estimands. For example, in a proof-of-concept study, focus may be solely on efficacy. However, as development progresses, focus may shift toward effectiveness.

Importantly, the choice of estimand influences study design. For example, focus on effectiveness implies more naturalistic settings, whereas focus on efficacy implies more highly controlled settings. Estimand 1 requires collection of follow-up data. Estimand 6 requires either follow-up data with no rescue medications or imputation of follow-up data. Estimand 2 requires a run-in phase.

The choice of the primary estimand also influences the choice of the primary analysis. Estimands 4 and 5 yield no missing data. Hence, no missing data assumptions are required and simple analytic approaches are appropriate. Estimands 2 and 3 require validity of MAR. Hence, many simple analytic methods and means of dealing with missing data will not be appropriate.

Estimands 1 and 6 allow for changes in treatment. With estimand 1, the analysis does not need to consider the treatment change because inference is on the treatment regimen. However, estimand 6 requires an analysis that can account for the change in treatments because inference is on the originally randomized medication.

The interactions between estimands, choice of data, study design, and data analyses highlights the need for cross-disciplinary discussions when considering how to prevent and treat missing data.

The Analytic Road Map

12.1 Introduction

The previous chapter illustrated estimands and common analytic approaches to estimate them. No matter how careful the choice of estimand and analysis, assumptions about the missing data are hard to avoid and it is important to understand the robustness of inferences to the assumptions. Such assessments can be made using sensitivity analyses.

Principles and methods for sensitivity analyses that quantify the robustness of inferences to departures from underlying assumptions is an emerging area of statistical science.

Because it is an active area of research, consensus does not exist on exactly how sensitivity analyses should be conducted and interpreted. However, the recent NRC guidance on prevention and treatment of missing data set forth principles and described methods consistent with those principles (NRC, 2010). The ideas presented in the NRC guidance are largely consistent with proposals and general ideas from Molenberghs and Kenward (2007) and Mallinckrodt et al. (2008). The methods and principles outlined in this chapter are a consolidated view of these recent recommendations.

Fundamental issues exist in selecting a model and assessing its fit to incomplete data that do not apply to inferences from complete data. While these issues occur in MAR analyses, they are compounded under MNAR. When the primary analysis assumes MAR, several aspects of the model fit can often be addressed by standard model-checking diagnostics. For example, it is possible to objectively evaluate distributional assumptions of the observed data, but, of course, distributional assumptions for the unobserved data cannot be directly assessed.

It is also possible in the MAR setting to assess the influence of individual or clusters of outlying observations on various aspects of model fit, as well as identifying observations that may be driving weakly identified parts of an MNAR model (Molenberghs and Kenward, 2007). Because it is not possible to determine the validity of MAR, sensitivity analyses are needed to assess how departures from MAR may impact results.

While this chapter covers distributional assumptions and influential observations, the focus is on sensitivity to assumptions about the missing data mechanism. This chapter begins by setting forth an overall analytic road map – a framework from which primary analyses and sensitivity analyses can be developed.

12.2 The Analytic Road Map

Even though the assumption of MAR is reasonable in many clinical trial scenarios, the possibility of MNAR cannot be excluded. It is tempting then to consider an MNAR method for the primary analysis. However, going beyond MAR to MNAR can only be done by making assumptions (Mallinckrodt et al., 2008). Conclusions from the MNAR analyses hinge on the appropriateness of those assumptions (Verbeke and Molenberghs, 2000). Because the data about which the assumptions are made is missing, MNAR analyses entail unverifiable assumptions (Laird, 1994). Importantly, the consequences of model misspecification are more severe with MNAR methods than with other (e.g., MAR) methods (Little, 1995; Laird, 1994; Rubin, 1994; Draper, 1995, Kenward, 1998). Hence, no individual MNAR analysis can be considered definitive.

Simply put, the conundrum missing data pose is that MCAR is usually not a reasonable assumption, MAR may be reasonable but there is no way to know for certain, and there is no way to be certain that an MNAR analysis is appropriate.

A sensible compromise between blindly shifting to MNAR models and ignoring them altogether is to use MNAR methods in sensitivity analyses (Molenberghs and Kenward, 2007; Mallinckrodt et al., 2008).

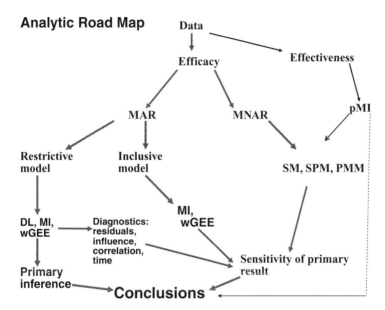

Figure 12.1. An analytic road map for continuous endpoints in longitudinal clinical trials.

Indeed, broad consensus has emerged indicating that the primary analyses of longitudinal clinical trials with continuous endpoints should often be based on methods that assume MAR, and that robustness of the MAR result should be assessed using sensitivity analyses (Verbeke and Molenberghs, 2000; Molenberghs and Kenward, 2007; Mallinckrodt et al., 2008; Siddiqui, Hung, and O'Neill, 2009).

To fix ideas developed in subsequent sections, Figure 12.1 depicts an analytic road map. A road map is different from driving directions. Unlike driving directions, a road map does not chart a specific, single course, with instructions on exactly how far to go and when to turn. Instead, the road map lays out the alternatives in a coherent manner such that the best route for a particular situation can be chosen.

Given that there is no universally best analytic approach, researchers are best served by understanding the alternatives rather than to be instructed what their choice should be in each of the myriad situations they may face. Therefore, the road map is not intended to be an all-encompassing prescription for all scenarios. Rather, it is specific to the example data analyzed in Chapter 14, but also provides a general framework that can be adapted to other scenarios.

As first outlined in Chapter 1, the goal is to specify as the primary analysis a "sensible" analysis. In this context, Carpenter and Kenward (2007) defined sensible as an analysis where:

1) The variation between the intervention effect estimated from patients in the trial and that in the population is random. In other words, trial results are not systematically biased in one direction.
2) As the sample size increases, the variation between the intervention effect estimated from patients in the trial and that in the population gets smaller and smaller. In other words, as the size of the trial increases, the estimated intervention effect hones in on the true value in the population. Such estimates are called *consistent* in statistical terminology.
3) The estimate of the variability between the trial intervention effect and the true effect in the population (i.e., the standard error) is accurate, and therefore correctly reflects the uncertainty in the data.

If all these conditions hold, then valid inference can be drawn despite the missing data.

12.3 Testable Assumptions

Standard Diagnostics

Important assumptions required for valid regression-type analyses of continuous outcomes include linearity, normality, and independence (Wonnacott and Wonnacott, 1981). These assumptions are in regards to the residuals (difference between observed and predicted values), not on the actual observations. These are standard statistical assumptions with no special considerations for missing data, except as noted previously, that departures from assumed distributions can be more problematic in MNAR models.

Therefore, rather than a detailed discussion of topics already well established in the literature, an illustration is provided in Chapter 14 of assessing the impact of correlation assumptions and potentially aberrant residuals on the effects of primary interest, such as the endpoint treatment contrast. This approach focuses not as much on whether or not deviations from the assumptions existed, but rather on how much (if at all) departures from assumptions influenced results. For example, if the residuals were not normally distributed, but this lack of normality had a trivial impact on the primary treatment contrast, then the result would be useful, even if not entirely valid in the strictest sense, because inferences were not contingent on this assumption.

Influence Diagnostics

Although methods to test for the existence and impact of outlier (influential) observations have been around for decades, new methods have been developed for use in MNAR analyses. To this end, interest has grown in local influence approaches (Shen et al., 2006; Zhu and Lee, 2001; Verbeke et al., 2001; Thijs, Molenberghs, and Verbeke, 2000; Molenberghs et al., 2001; Troxel, Ma, and Heitjan, 2004; Ma, Troxel, and Heitjan, 2005), which are often associated with selection models. Local influence provides an objective approach to identifying and examining the impact of influential observations and clusters of observations on various aspects of the analysis, including the missing-data mechanisms and treatment effects.

However, given the newness and complexity of such methods, and that key principles do not markedly differ from simpler methods, the key points are illustrated using simpler methods in Chapter 14. These simpler methods enjoy the benefit of being implementable using standard, commercially available software. The basic idea is again not to simply identify if or if not influential observations were present, but rather to assess how the most influential observations influenced the parameters of primary interest.

12.4 Assessing Sensitivity to Missing Data Assumptions

It was previously mentioned in Chapter 2 and elsewhere that the assumption of MCAR is unlikely to hold in most clinical trial scenarios. It is possible to objectively assess the validity of MCAR. For example, in a logistic regression analysis of probability of dropout, if the primary efficacy variable was associated with the probability of dropout, then MCAR did not hold for this outcome. In addition, tests can be conducted to compare visitwise means for patients that dropped out versus patients that continued. If means are not equal, there is strong evidence to reject MCAR.

Assessing the validity of MAR is a different matter because, as previously noted, the characteristics that differentiate MAR from MNAR involve the missing data. The focus of sensitivity analyses should be on sensitivity to assumptions, not sensitivity to methods. Many methods (e.g., likelihood-based mixed models, multiple imputation, EM algorithm, among others) rely on the same assumption: that data are MAR. Therefore, comparing results from these methods does not assess sensitivity to the assumption of MAR and could lead to a misleadingly optimistic view of the robustness of the conclusions.

Another example would be to use a likelihood-based analysis as primary and then use LOCF or BOCF as a sensitivity analysis. Given the historical precedent for LOCF and BOCF, there may be a certain confidence engendered by seeing results from LOCF and BOCF. However, that confidence would be largely misplaced given that LOCF and BOCF do not provide information about the validity of MAR in a likelihood-based analysis. Instead, sensitivity analyses need to vary the assumptions, and then use appropriate techniques to estimate the effect of the intervention under these alternative assumptions. The aim is to establish how robust the estimates are to such alternatives.

In a broad sense, sensitivity analyses can be defined as one in which several statistical models are considered simultaneously – or in which a statistical model is further scrutinized using specialized tools, such as diagnostic measures (NRC, 2010). A simple procedure is to fit a selected number of models, all of which are deemed plausible. The degree to which conclusions (inferences) are stable across such analyses provides an indication of the confidence that can be placed in them.

The focus should be on comparing the magnitude of the primary treatment contrasts from the various sensitivity analyses with that from the primary analysis. Emphasis should not be placed heavily on p values as this can be misleading. For example, assume the primary result from an MAR analysis with a restrictive model yielded a p value of .049.

Further assume that the assumption of MAR for this primary analysis was valid. When moving to inclusive models, the additional variables will have no additional predictive value because the primary analysis fully accounted for the dropout. However, given more variables are being fit in the analysis, the standard error will likely increase, thereby increasing the p value to greater than .05.

Simply tallying up the number of significant and non-significant results across the set of sensitivity analyses would likely see most p values cross the line to non-significance, resulting in the erroneous conclusion that the primary result was not robust to the MAR assumption. In contrast, emphasizing the magnitude of the treatment contrast would in this situation show consistent results, thereby correctly implying the results were robust to departures from MAR.

A logical place to begin sensitivity analyses is to implement a more inclusive model for the MAR-based primary analysis. Recall that in Chapter 7 inclusive models were introduced as models that, in addition to the design factors of the experiment that are the focus in restrictive models, auxiliary variables that are potentially predictive of dropout, are added to the model. This can change a missing data mechanism that would have otherwise been MNAR into MAR.

The next step in sensitivity can be to implement a series of plausible MNAR analyses. In so doing, one approach in the MNAR framework is to estimate from the available data the parameters of a model representing a plausible MNAR mechanism. However, the data typically do not contain information on the MNAR parameters of such models (Jansen et al., 2006b). In fact, different MNAR models may fit the observed data equally well but have quite different implications for the unobserved measurements and hence for the conclusions to be drawn from the respective analyses (Molenberghs and Kenward, 2007).

Therefore, in addition to estimating the MNAR parameters, which is driven by assumption, it is useful to vary the parameters describing the MNAR mechanism across a plausible range. For example, a selection model can be implemented in which from the dropout model an estimate of the association between the present, possibly missing efficacy outcome and the probability of dropout is obtained. However, it is hard to have confidence in this estimate. Therefore, subsequent selection models can be run wherein differing values of this parameter are input and fixed in the analysis, thereby facilitating assessment of changes in the magnitude of the primary treatment contrast across the various analyses.

Similarly, various pattern mixture and shared-parameter models can be fit. For example, pattern mixture models with varying but plausible identifying restrictions can be fit and compared, or shared-parameter models with increasingly complex linkages between the measurement and dropout models can be fit and compared.

Depending on the primary estimand, controlled imputation approaches hold promise as sensitivity analyses. Analyses in these frameworks can be formulated to tailor control of the distributional assumptions for specific purposes. For example, imputations can be controlled to yield a conservative but principled estimate of the treatment contrast, thereby creating a floor value for what Molenberghs and Kenward (2007) refer to as the interval or region of ignorance.

For example, in the acute, symptomatic treatment of depression example examined in Chapter 14, the pMI approach is implemented under the assumption that, conditional on previous outcomes, the distribution of both drug- and placebo-treated patients after discontinuation of study drug is that of placebo patients. For a primary efficacy estimand, this analysis is likely biased toward the null hypothesis of no difference between treatments. The estimate from such an analysis could therefore be considered the worst reasonable case result. If the treatment effect from such an analysis was satisfactorily large, it could be safely concluded that a treatment effect existed. The other sensitivity analyses would likely yield less conservative estimates.

12.5 Considerations

The wide range of models and methods for handling missing data highlights the need for sensitivity analysis. Emphasis on sensitivity analyses is shifting from what had been ever-more complex approaches to those with more transparent and easily debated and manipulated assumptions.

Although consensus does not exist on how to draw inferences in a sensitivity framework, recent guidance provides clarity on a number of methods and principles. While there will always be need for sensitivity analyses inspired by trial results, a parsimonious set of logical and plausible sensitivity analyses should be prespecified.

The ideas presented in this chapter and reinforced in the example in Chapter 14 are not meant to be prescriptive as to how every sensitivity analysis should be conducted, but rather to illustrate general principles that can guide practice. As the clinical contexts vary between studies, so too should the specific form of the sensitivity analyses (NRC, 2010). In particular, the extent of the sensitivity analyses is dictated by the diversity in assumptions that are plausible.

Analyzing Incomplete Categorical Data

13.1 Introduction

Many of the principles regarding analysis of incomplete data previously discussed for continuous outcomes also apply to categorical outcomes. For example, the missing data mechanisms (Chapter 2) apply to categorical data in essentially the same manner as for continuous data. In addition, considerations regarding modeling time and correlation are also essentially the same as previously outlined for continuous outcomes (Chapter 7). As with continuous data, likelihood-based methods are appealing because of their flexible ignorability properties (Chapter 8). However, their use for categorical outcomes can be problematic because of increased computational requirements as compared with continuous data. Therefore, GEE is a useful alternative.

Despite the similarities between continuous and categorical analyses of incomplete data, some aspects are unique to categorical outcomes, and that is the focus of this chapter. The next section begins with a discussion on marginal and conditional inference because this sets the stage for subsequent sections that discuss the similarities and differences between analyses of continuous and categorical data.

13.2 Marginal and Conditional Inference

To illustrate marginal and conditional inference, consider the probability of developing a certain disease. Let D be a discrete random variable taking on a value of 1 for subjects with the disease and 0 if not. Let T be a discrete random variable describing the probability of having 0, 1, or 2 risk factors for the disease. Further assume that the probabilities of D depend on T. That is, $P(D = 1)$ and $P(D = 0)$ vary depending on whether T is 0, 1, or 2. With $T = 2$ (two risk factors), $P(D = 1)$ is greater than if $T = 1$, and $P(D = 1)$ is greater when $T = 1$ than if $T = 0$. Hypothetical data for the example are listed below.

	Joint Distribution: $P(D,T)$			
	$T = 0$	$T = 1$	$T = 2$	Marginal Probability
D = 0 (healthy)	0.693	0.09	0.04	0.823
D = 1 (disease)	0.007	0.01	0.16	0.177
Total	0.7	0.1	0.2	1

Finding the probability for specific pairs of outcomes, D and T, requires knowledge of the joint probability distribution. An example would be the probability of a patient having both $D = 1$ and $T = 0$, which in this example is .007. That is, 0.7% of the sample developed the disease *and* had 0 risk factors.

An example of marginal inference from these data would be questions about the probability of D without regard for T. The marginal $P(D = 1)$ can be found by summing the probabilities for $D = 1$ across all levels of T. In the example, the marginal $P(D = 1) = .007 + .01 + .16 = .177$. The marginal $P(D = 0)$ can be found similarly by summing across all levels of T where $D = 0$ (.823 in the example).

An example of conditional inference from these data would be questions about the probability of D at specific values of T. For example, what is the probability of getting the disease for patients with one risk factor? From the preceding table, if $T = 1$ (one risk factor), the probability $D = 1$ (disease) $= .01$ and the probability $D = 0$ (healthy) $= .09$. The conditional probability is based on only those patients with $T = 1$. Hence, the probability $D = 1$ given $T = 1$ (which can be denoted as $p(D = 1|T = 1) = .01 / (.01 + .09) = 10\%$. Similarly, the $P(D = 1|T = 2$ is calculated as $.16 / (.16 + .04) = 80\%$.

None of these three inferential frameworks (joint, marginal, and conditional) is inherently more relevant than the others; each can be the most relevant or not relevant at all depending on the question being addressed.

The distinctions between marginal and conditional inference are relevant in longitudinal trials of medical interventions, but perhaps not as straightforward as in the previous simplistic example. Consider a situation in which an outcome variable Y is to be analyzed for i subjects at j measurement times.

In marginal models, marginal distributions are used to describe the outcome vector Y, given a set of X predictor variables. The correlation among the components of Y (e.g., repeated measurements taken over time on the same subjects) can then be captured either via a fully parametric approach (as in likelihood-based analyses) or by working assumptions (as in the semi-parametric GEE approach). In a random-effects model, the predictor variables in X are supplemented with a vector of random effects, conditional on which the components of Y are usually assumed to be independent, although residual dependence can still be accommodated. Finally, a conditional model describes the distribution of the components of Y, conditional on X and conditional on (a subset of) the other components of Y.

Although statistical notation has been used sparingly, the following examples use such notation because it is can make understanding key points easier. A marginal model for normally distributed data starts by specifying

$$E(Y_{ij}|X_{ij}) = X'_{ij}\beta. \tag{13.1}$$

That is, the expected value of outcome variable Y on subject i at measurement occasion j is equal to a set of fixed effects, such as treatment group, baseline predictors, and so on. Marginal inference is carried out by analyzing Y with respect to the fixed effects that are included in X, the solutions to which are in β.

In a random-effects model, the focus is on the expectation, conditional on the random-effects vector. That is, to the previous fixed effects, random effects (b_i) are added:

$$E(Y_{ij}|x_{ij}, b_i) = x'_{ij}\beta + z'_{ij}b_i. \tag{13.2}$$

The conditional model uses expectations of the form

$$E(Y_{ij}|Y_{i,j-1}, \ldots, Y_{i1}, x_{ij}) = x'_{ij}\beta + \alpha Y_{i,j-1}. \tag{13.3}$$

That is, rather than add random effects as in Equation (13.2), expectations are based on previous observations.

In linear mixed model analyses of continuous outcomes, the elegant properties of the normal distribution imply a simple marginal model if a random-effects model is used. Specifically, the expectation (13.1) follows from (13.3) either by marginalizing over the random effects or by conditioning on the random-effects vector $b_i = 0$.

Therefore, for normally distributed data, the fixed-effects parameters ß, which include treatment effects, have both a marginal and a hierarchical model interpretation. The conditional models are less useful in the context of longitudinal clinical trial data (Molenberghs and Verbeke, 2005). Specifically, interest is most often on an overall, or population average treatment effect, not on a treatment effect associated with a specific outcome history. Therefore, conditional models will not be further considered here.

Given the connection between marginal and random-effects models, it is clear why the linear mixed model provides a unifying framework for the analysis of continuous data. This connection between the model families does not exist when outcomes are non-normal, such as binary, categorical, or discrete (Jansen et al., 2006a). Therefore, marginal and random-effects models in the context of categorical data are considered in detail.

Thorough discussions on marginal modeling can be found in Diggle, Heagerty, Liang, and Zeger (2002) and in Fahrmeir and Tutz (2001). The specific context of clustered binary data has received treatment in Aerts, Geys, Molenberghs and Ryan (2002).

13.3 Generalized Estimating Equations

Generalized estimating equations can circumvent the computational complexity of likelihood-based analyses of categorical data, and therefore represent a viable alternative whenever interest is restricted to the mean parameters (treatment difference, time evolutions, effect of baseline covariates, etc.). In GEE, the missing data mechanism must be MCAR in order to be ignorable. Hence, similar to continuous data, weighted generalized estimating equations have been proposed to extend ignorability to both MCAR and MAR (see Chapter 9 for more details).

Generalized estimating equations are rooted in the quasi-likelihood ideas expressed by McCullagh and Nelder (1989). Modeling is restricted to the correct specification of the marginal mean function, together with so-called working assumptions about the correlation structure among the repeated measures.

As detailed in Chapter 9, GEE is valid only under MCAR, hence the interest in weighted GEE. With categorical data, as with continuous data, the idea is to weight each subject's contribution in the GEEs by the inverse probability that a subject drops out at the time of dropout. Hence in practice, the only major modification needed for wGEE of categorical data compared with continuous data is to account for the difference in distributions, which can be done by specifying a link function for the means and an appropriate distribution for the residuals. For binary data, the logit link is a common choice. That is, rather than analyze the binary (0 / 1) data, the logit transformation is applied and the logits are analyzed.

In GEE analyses, empirical standard errors are larger than the model-based standard errors because model-based standard errors are the ones that would be obtained if the estimating equations were true likelihood equations – that is, when the working correlation structure is correct. In such cases likelihood inference is optimal. However, given that the working correlation structure is allowed to be misspecified in wGEE, model-based standard errors will be biased and it is advisable to base conclusions on empirically corrected standard errors – that is, the so-called sandwich estimator should be used (Jansen et al., 2006a).

13.4 Random-Effects Models

Unlike correlated Gaussian outcomes, the parameters of the random-effects and population-averaged (marginal) models for correlated binary data describe different types of effects of the covariates on the response probabilities (Jansen et al., 2006a). Therefore, the choice between population-averaged (marginal) and random-effects models depends on the scientific goals.

Population-averaged models evaluate the categorical outcome as a function of covariates only. With a subject-specific approach, the response is modeled as a function of covariates and parameters specific to each subject. In such models, interpretation of fixed-effects parameters is conditional on the random effects. That is, with random effects models for categorical data, inferences about the treatment effect do not apply to the population as a whole; they apply to the sample of patients analyzed. Again, with continuous data this problem does not exist because of the interchangeability arising from the properties of the normal distribution.

A general formulation of mixed-effects models was given by Jansen et al. (2006a) as follows. Assume that $\mathbf{Y}_i$ (possibly appropriately transformed) satisfies

$$Y_i|b_i \sim F_i(\theta, b_i). \tag{13.4}$$

That is, conditional on $\mathbf{b}_i$, $\mathbf{Y}_i$ follows a prespecified distribution F_i, possibly depending on covariates and parameterized through a vector θ of unknown parameters common to all subjects. Furthermore $\mathbf{b}_i$ is a q-dimensional vector of subject-specific parameters, called random effects, assumed to follow a so-called mixing distribution G, which may depend on a vector ψ of unknown parameters (i.e., $\mathbf{b}_i \sim G(\psi)$). The $\mathbf{b}_i$ reflects the between-unit heterogeneity in the population with respect to the distribution of $\mathbf{Y}_i$. In the presence of random effects, conditional independence is often assumed, under which the components Y_{ij} in $\mathbf{Y}_i$ are independent, conditional on $\mathbf{b}_i$. The distribution function F_i in Equation (13.4) is then a product of the n_i independent elements in $\mathbf{Y}_i$.

Generally, inference is based on the marginal model for $\mathbf{Y}_i$, obtained by integrating out the random effects over their distribution $G(\psi)$. This integration is where much of the additional complexity for analyses of categorical data is involved. Although the specific details of various analytic approaches, in particular the integrating out of the random effects, is important, the complexity of this topic is beyond our present focus. Jansen et al. (2006a) provided additional details. Recent developments in software tools are relevant to this topic, and statisticians should consult the most recent software releases for details. These software advances have allowed for more appropriate likelihood-based analyses that have replaced earlier approximations, thereby fostering greater correspondence between continuous and categorical analyses in the likelihood framework.

A formulation of the general linear mixed-effects model (GLMM) is as follows. Conditionally on random effects b_i, it is assumed that the elements Y_{ij} of $\mathbf{Y}_i$ are independent, with density function usually based on a classical exponential family formulation, that is, with mean

$$E(Y_{ij}|\mathbf{b}_i) = a'(\eta_{ij}) = \boldsymbol{\mu}_{ij}(\mathbf{b}_i) \text{ and variance } Var(Y_{ij}|bi) = \varphi a''(\eta_{ij}),$$

(13.5)

and where, apart from a link function h (e.g., the logit link for binary data or the poisson link for counts), a linear regression model with parameters β and $\mathbf{b}_i$ is used for the mean

$$h(\boldsymbol{\mu}_i(\mathbf{b}_i)) = X_i \text{ß} + Z_i \mathbf{b}_i.$$

(13.6)

Note that the linear mixed model for continuous data is a special case of this model with an identity link function. The random effects $\mathbf{b}_i$ are again assumed to be sampled from a (multivariate) normal distribution with mean $\mathbf{0}$ and covariance matrix D. Usually, the canonical link function is used, that is, $h = a'^{-1}$, such that $\eta_i = Xi\beta + Z_i\mathbf{b}_i$. With a logit link and normally distributed random effects, the familiar logistic-linear GLMM follows.

13.5 Multiple Imputation

Another method for analyses of categorical incomplete data is to use multiple imputation to impute the missing values, followed by an analytic approach that would have been suitable had the data been complete (Schafer, 2003). See Chapter 8 for basic details of multiple imputation and Chapter 9 for specific examples of MI for continuous data.

Multiple imputation can be especially straightforward and useful for the analyses of dichotomized continuous variables. For example, assume that in the hypothetical data first presented in Table 9.1, a change from baseline of 30% is used as the cutoff to define clinically meaningful improvement. Each efficacy response on the original, continuous scale is categorized as clinically meaningful improvement yes/no.

Imputations could proceed to fill in the missing binary, yes/no outcome. However, given the loss of information from dichotomizing continuous outcomes, it may be preferable to impute the missing values on the continuous scale and then categorize all outcomes, both observed and imputed, as meeting the criteria for response yes or no.

Although the specific details go beyond the present scope, when imputing missing values on the categorical scale, attention to distributional assumptions inherent to the specific method of imputation can be important. For a discussion of these issues, see Schafer (2003).

13.6 Considerations

Methods used to account for missing continuous data also apply to categorical data. For example, wGEE, likelihood-based mixed-effects models, and multiple imputation are all valid under MAR. Modeling considerations for time and correlation are also similar to the continuous data case.

However, unlike in the continuous case where the linear mixed model is the main analytic tool, for categorical data, analysts much choose between a marginal model (e.g., generalized estimating equations, GEE) and a random-effects approach (generalized linear mixed models, GLMM). These approaches may provide similar results in terms of hypothesis testing for treatment effects. However, for estimation purposes, the model differences are important because the parameters have different meanings.

14

Example

14.1 Introduction

This chapter illustrates via retrospective analyses of a longitudinal clinical trial how the principles and recommendations outlined in previous chapters can be applied a priori, such as would be required in regulatory settings for confirmatory trials and for optimum decision making in early phase trials. The next section describes the setting, the data, and the originally reported results from the trial used in the present re-analysis. Section 14.3 specifies the objectives and Section 14.4 describes the analysis plan for the retrospective analyses as they could be prespecified, using ideas presented in Chapter 12. The results from the retrospective analyses are presented in Section 14.5, followed by a discussion on how principled inferences can be drawn from the results.

Having proper tools to conduct sensitivity analyses is essential if they are to be a routine part of clinical trial analysis and reporting. Software tools to implement the various analyses presented in this chapter are made available in Chapter 15.

14.2 Data and Setting

A clinical trial in major depressive disorder, originally reported by Detke et al. (2002), is used for the present illustration. This trial compared the efficacy of an experimental antidepressant with placebo to support a New Drug Application. As such, this was a phase III (confirmatory) trial. Patients were randomly assigned (1:1 ratio) to placebo (n = 139) or the experimental drug (n = 128), with the double-blind treatment period lasting 9 weeks. Study visits were scheduled once a week for the first 3 weeks after randomization, and every 2 weeks thereafter.

The experimental drug was significantly superior to placebo on the a priori declared primary efficacy analysis (likelihood-based repeated measures) of mean change to endpoint on the 17-item Hamilton rating scale for depression ($HAMD_{17}$) total score ($p = 0.025$). The completion rates were 64.7% for placebo and 60.9% for the experimental drug. The rates of dropout attributable to adverse events were 4.3% for placebo and 12.5% for the experimental drug, while the corresponding rates of dropout attributable to lack of efficacy were 13.7% and 5.5%, respectively.

Although results were significant based on the primary analysis, it was reasonable to wonder to what degree missing data might have biased the estimate of treatment efficacy. As was customary at the time, detailed sensitivity analyses were not included in the primary reporting of this trial.

14.3 Objectives and Estimands

For the present re-analysis it was important to understand both efficacy and effectiveness – that is, the treatment effect when the drug was taken as directed and what happened as the drug was actually taken. Therefore, the re-analysis included tests of both de jure (efficacy) and de facto (effectiveness) hypotheses. Estimands were discussed in Chapter 3 and further consideration of how choice of estimand influences choice of analysis were covered in Chapter 11. The overall plan for re-analysis is depicted in Figure 12.1, the analytic road map.

The primary focus of the re-analysis, as for the original analysis, was on efficacy. Specifically the primary objective was to compare drug versus control in the mean change from baseline to the planned endpoint (Visit 8, Week 9) expected if patients stayed in the study. The advantage of this efficacy estimand was that it fostered causal inference about the effects of the investigational drug. The disadvantage was that this estimand assessed a hypothetical treatment in that it is unrealistic to expect all patients will adhere to treatment. Nevertheless, it is important to understand what to expect when patients do adhere.

The secondary focus of the re-analysis was on effectiveness – that is, to compare drug versus control in mean change from baseline to the planned endpoint assuming that patients who discontinued study medication had less benefit from it than patients that adhered. The advantage of this effectiveness estimand was that it fostered causal inference for the investigational drug. The disadvantage was that this estimand was being applied to a double-blind trial of a medication that was not known to be safe and effective at the time the trial began. Therefore, patients and doctors likely made decisions about continuing treatment that would be different from the decisions made in a more naturalistic clinical setting.

The primary analysis for estimating the primary estimand was a likelihood-based approach using unstructured modeling of time and within-patient correlation, and random effects were modeled as part of the within-patient errors. Modeling considerations were covered in Chapter 7, Section 7.3.

Assumptions of the primary analysis for which sensitivity was assessed in the re-analysis included the assumption that missing data arose from an MAR mechanism. Robustness of results to the MAR assumption was assessed by comparing the magnitude of the treatment effect estimated from the primary (likelihood-based) analysis to the estimates obtained from various methods that assumed a missing not at random (MNAR) mechanism, and to other MAR methods that used inclusive models. Methods valid under MNAR were discussed in Chapter 10.

14.4 Analysis Plan

The following subsections describe the way the primary analysis and sensitivity analyses were implemented for this re-analysis. Similar verbiage could be used to prespecify analyses in study protocols and statistical analysis plans.

Primary Analysis

Mean changes from baseline were analyzed using a restricted maximum likelihood (REML)-based repeated measures approach. The analysis included the fixed, categorical effects of treatment, investigative site, visit, and treatment-by-visit interaction, as well as the continuous, fixed covariates of baseline score and baseline score-by-visit-interaction. An unstructured (co)variance structure was used to model the within-patient errors. The Kenward-Roger approximation was used to estimate denominator degrees of freedom and adjust standard errors. Significance tests were based on least-squares means using a two-sided $\alpha = 0.05$ (two-sided 95% confidence intervals). Analyses were implemented using SAS PROC MIXED (SAS, 2003). The primary comparison was the contrast between treatments at Visit 8, Week 9.

Prespecification of this analysis should also include provisions for the analysis failing to converge. In practice, failure to converge can often be attributable to issues in data preparation (Mallinckrodt et al., 2008). However, specifying an ever-more parsimonious set of plausible correlations structures to be tested if unstructured fails to converge is good practice. The primary analysis could be considered the first structure in the ever-more parsimonious set to yield convergence, or the structure yielding the best fit as measured by common model-fitting criteria (e.g., Akaike's information criterion). For confirmatory trials it has been more common to use the first-to-converge approach as this avoids model building and hypothesis testing from the same data, and it ensures the most general plausible structure is used.

Sensitivity to Correlation Assumptions

The validity of likelihood-based analyses hinges on correct specification of the correlation structure. Standard practice has moved to use of an unstructured correlation matrix for modeling the within-patient errors as a means of avoiding misspecification. However, this approach does not guarantee validity. For example, if the unstructured approach fails to converge, a more parsimonious model is likely necessary, but not necessarily correct. Moreover, structures more general than unstructured are possible, such as separate unstructured matrices by group (treatment).

Use of the sandwich estimator for standard errors in place of the model-based approach provides valid inference when the correlation structure is misspecified (Verbeke and Molenberghs, 2000). Therefore, use of the sandwich estimator as the default approach would protect against correlation misspecification. However, when the sandwich estimator is used in SAS PROC MIXED, only the between-within method for estimating denominator degrees of freedom is available, an approach that is known to be biased, especially in small samples. Moreover, the sandwich estimator assumes MCAR, which is difficult to justify a priori.

Therefore, an unstructured correlation matrix was used for the primary analysis, and a series of ever-more parsimonious structures was tested. Treatment contrasts from more general and more parsimonious structures, with and without use of the sandwich estimator, were compared. Results are summarized in Table 14.2.

Influence Diagnostics

The influence option (see Section 12.3) available in the model statement of SAS PROC MIXED (SAS, 2003) was used to determine which levels of clustering factors had the greatest influence on the primary analysis, focusing on impact to the endpoint treatment contrast. The clustering factors of interest were investigative site and patient. No specific cutoff was used to identify a site or patient as influential. Instead, natural breaks in the ascending sequence of Cook's D statistic (Cook and Weisberg, 1982) were used to determine cutoffs for identifying an effect as influential or not.

Sites with the greatest Cook's D statistic were excluded one at a time and the primary analysis repeated on each data subset. The endpoint treatment contrast from the primary analysis of the full data was compared to results with influential sites removed. Results are summarized in Table 14.3.

The same general process was used to assess influential patients. However, all patients identified as influential were deleted by treatment group rather than one at a time. The primary analysis was repeated with all influential drug-treated patients removed, with all influential placebo-treated patients removed, and with all influential patients removed. Results are summarized in Table 14.4.

The influence procedure as implemented in SAS PROC MIXED (SAS, 2003) is similar to a case deletion approach. Therefore, whichever effect is being diagnosed cannot be included in the fixed effects model as the case deletion alters the rank of the X matrix. Hence, when assessing the influence of sites, site was excluded from the model. This was not necessary when assessing the influence of patients as this effect was only in the within-in patient correlation structure, not in the fixed effects.

Residual Diagnostics

Observations with a studentized residual $> = 2.0$ or $= < -2.0$ were considered aberrant.

The primary analysis was repeated with all observations from drug-treated patients having aberrant residuals removed, with all observations from placebo-treated patients having aberrant residuals removed, and deleting all the observations having aberrant residuals. Results are summarized in Table 14.5.

Sensitivity to Missing Data Assumptions

The primary analysis utilized a restrictive model that included only the design factors of the experiment, and assumed missing data arose from a missing at random (MAR) mechanism. Therefore, the focus of missing data sensitivity analyses was on expanding the scope of MAR by including additional variables potentially predictive of dropout in an inclusive modeling framework and on using a variety of MNAR methods that relied on differing but plausible assumptions. Inclusive models were implemented within the wGEE and multiple imputation frameworks. This was done so that both methods could be illustrated. In practice, there would be a need to use only one of these methods as they both rely on the same assumptions. In addition, MNAR analyses were implemented within the selection model, shared-parameter model, and pattern-mixture model frameworks, including controlled imputation.

In the wGEE analyses, the probability of dropout for each patient at each visit, given the patient was observed at the previous visit, was estimated and the probabilities were accumulated over visits. The probability of dropout was modeled using logistic regression via PROC GENMOD in SAS (SAS, 2003) using a logit link and binary errors. The model for analyzing dropout included treatment, the primary outcome variable ($HAMD_{17}$ total score), visit, patient-rated global impression of improvement (PGI), clinician-rated global impression of improvement (CGI), and all two-way interactions between covariates and treatment.

The inverse probabilities from the logistic regression were used to weight the observations for the analyses of the outcome variable. Weighted analyses of the outcome variable were conducted in PROC

GENMOD (SAS, 2003) using an identity link and normally distributed errors.

Multiple imputation with an inclusive model was implemented using the SAS PROC MI and PROC MI ANALYZE (SAS, 2003). Imputation models included the previous outcomes of the dependent variable plus the same auxiliary variables as included in the wGEE analysis. The resulting completed data sets were analyzed with direct likelihood as implemented for the primary analysis. Results from the completed data sets were combined and inferences were drawn according to Rubin's rules (Rubin, 1987). Results from inclusive modeling are summarized in Table 14.6.

A parametric version of the selection model was implemented in SAS using PROC MIXED for relevant analyses and starting values and PROC IML to build and solve necessary equations and evaluate likelihoods. The continuous outcome (change from baseline in $HAMD_{17}$ total score) was modeled using the same fixed-effects and correlation structure as for the primary analysis. The log odds for probability of dropout were modeled in the logistic regression part of the model using previous and current, possibly unobserved, primary efficacy outcomes, treatment, and the interaction of primary efficacy outcome with treatment.

In addition to an analysis where all parameters were estimated, various values for the regression parameters that assessed the relationship between the possibly missing current observation and the probability of dropout were assumed in order to assess robustness of the endpoint treatment contrast across a wide range of MNAR conditions, as assumed to exist in a selection model. Fixing the regression coefficients at 0 assumed MAR. Selection model results are summarized in Table 14.7.

For the pattern-mixture model analyses, patients were assigned to groups defined as early dropout, late dropout, or completer. The identifying restrictions used were non-future-dependent, complete case missing value (NFD_CCMV) and non-future-dependent, neighboring case missing value (NFD_MCMV). Pattern-mixture model results are summarized in Table 14.8.

For the shared-parameter model analyses, the intent was to model the primary outcome using the same fixed-effects and correlation structure as for the primary analysis, and to use the primary efficacy outcome in the time to event portion of the analysis. However, given that numeric difficulties can arise in these more complex models, simplified models were implemented. For example, a parametric model for time that included linear and quadratic components was used rather than a fully unstructured model, and investigative site was not included in the model.

Several versions with progressively more complex linkages between the measurement and dropout models were implemented using SAS PROC NLMIXED (SAS, 2003). The first model had no linkage between the measurement and dropout models. Model 2 included random intercept and slope terms for the measurement and dropout models, and Model 3 added additional interaction terms for separate intercepts and slopes by treatment group. The primary treatment contrasts from these models were compared to assess the potential impact of departures from MAR as assumed in a shared-parameter model. Shared-parameter model results are summarized in Table 14.9.

Placebo multiple imputation was used both as an assessment of effectiveness and as a worst reasonable case assessment of efficacy. To implement this approach, multiple imputation was used to replace missing outcomes for both drug-treated and placebo-treated patients who discontinued using multiple draws from the posterior predictive distribution estimated from patients who were randomized to placebo. The imputation model included changes from baseline in the primary efficacy outcome. The endpoint contrast and associated confidence interval and p values were obtained from the multiple datasets using Rubin's rules (Rubin, 1987, p. 75), as implemented in SAS PROC MI ANALYZE (SAS, 2003). Results from pMI are summarized in Table 14.10.

14.5 Results

Descriptive Statistics and Graphs

The first step in analysis is to understand the data. Even in situations where analysis plans are based on abundant historical data, it is necessary to understand the data in hand. Although a number of graphical and summary approaches are needed to fully understand the breadth of the data, focus here is on missing data.

Table 14.1. *Visitwise Means for Completers and Patients that Discontinued Treatment Early*

Week	Therapy	Number Continuing	Continuers' Mean	Number Dropping	Dropouts' Mean
1	Drug	110	−2.8	13	−2.9
1	Placebo	129	−2.7	7	−1.1
2	Drug	107	−5.4	2	−3.5
2	Placebo	122	−4.5	7	−4.1
3	Drug	98	−6.7	10	−6.9
3	Placebo	111	−6.1	11	−6.0
5	Drug	89	−8.9	9	−3.4
5	Placebo	97	−8.2	14	−1.0
7	Drug	81	−10.4	8	−10.0
7	Placebo	90	−8.6	7	−7.1
9	Drug	81	−10.7		
9	Placebo	90	−9.0		

Time to treatment discontinuation is summarized in Figure 14.1. The drug group had more discontinuations early in the trial, but the gap between treatments was reduced over time. Tables 14.1 and Figure 14.2 provide information on differences between patients that completed the trial versus those who discontinued treatment early. These data show that patients who discontinued early tended to have less favorable efficacy outcomes than completers, and were particularly prone to discontinue after a worsening in response. Combining this evidence with the rates of discontinuations attributable to lack of efficacy provided strong evidence that missing data for the primary outcome did not arise from an MCAR mechanism.

Correlation, Influence, and Residual Diagnostics

Results from analyses of the primary outcome using various correlation structures are summarized in Table 14.2. These results showed that an unstructured correlation matrix provided the best fit. Robustness of results was further confirmed in that the treatment effect was consistent across the various structures.

Results from analyses of the primary outcome excluding influential sites are summarized in Table 14.3. Sites 999, 115, and 122 were the most influential sites. Deleting sites 999 and 115 increased the magnitude of

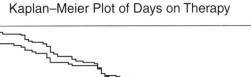

Kaplan–Meier Plot of Days on Therapy

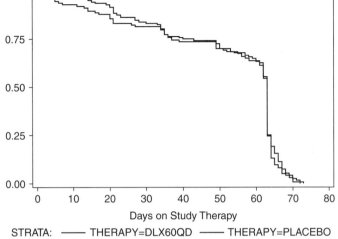

Figure 14.1. Kaplan-Meier plot of days on treatment.

Visitwise Mean Change From Baseline for Completers and Dropouts at Each Visit by Therapy

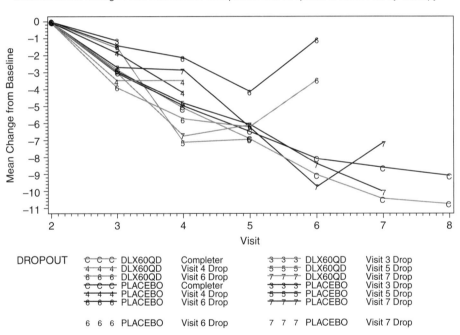

Figure 14.2. Visitwise means for completers and for patients who discontinued treatment early.

Table 14.2. *Results from Varying Correlation Structures in Likelihood-Based Analyses of the Primary Outcome*

Correlation Structure	Grouping[1]	Standard Error Method	AIC Model Fit	Endpoint Contrast	Standard Error
Unstructured	Overall	Sandwich	7,273.42	−2.16	0.931
Unstructured	Overall	Model-based	7,273.42	−2.16	0.957
Unstructured	By drug	Model-based	7,290.51	−2.11	0.953
TOEPH[2]	Overall	Model-based	7,293.54	−2.08	0.893
TOEPH	By drug	Model-based	7,297.73	−2.08	0.894
CSH[3]	Overall	Model-based	7,441.55	−2.32	0.926
CSH	By drug	Model-based	7,448.86	−2.32	0.919

[1] Overall = one correlation for all patients. By drug = separate correlation structures for each treatment.
[2] TOEPH = Heterogeneous Toeplitz
[3] CSH = Heterogeneous compound symmetric

the treatment effect, while deleting site 122 resulted in a small reduction to the treatment effect. Therefore, the estimated treatment effect was not driven by a single site.

Results from analyses of the primary outcome excluding influential patients are summarized ion Table 14.4. Dropping placebo- and drug-treated influential patients both increased the magnitude of the treatment effect, with the difference being more pronounced when dropping influential placebo-treated patients. The 6 influential placebo-treated patients tended to have large responses, whereas the responses for the 2 influential drug-treated patients were on average similar to the sample as a whole. As expected from a large, confirmatory trial, the treatment effects was not driven by one or a few subjects.

Table 14.3. *Results from the Primary Outcome with Data from Influential Sites Excluded*

Dataset	Number of Patients	Number of Observations	Endpoint Contrast
All Sites	259	1,293	−2.16
Drop Site 999	194	960	−2.40
Drop Site 115	198	974	−2.56
Drop Site 122	211	1,093	−2.06

Table 14.4. *Results from the Primary Outcome with Data from Influential Patients Excluded*

Dataset	Number of Patients	Number of Observations	Endpoint Contrast
All Data	259	1,293	−2.16
DropPlacebo	252	1,253	−2.62
DropDrug	257	1,286	−2.20
DropAll	250	1,246	−2.67

Results from analyses of the primary outcome excluding patients with aberrant residuals are summarized in Table 14.5. Excluding placebo-treated patients with aberrant residuals decreased the magnitude of the treatment effect by approximately 10%. Excluding drug-treated patients with aberrant residuals had minimal impact on the magnitude of the treatment contrast. The distribution of the residuals was symmetric and did not markedly differ from the assumed normal distribution.

Missing Data Sensitivity Analyses

Results from inclusive modeling wGEE and MI analyses of the primary outcome are summarized in Table 14.6. The inclusive model analyses yielded endpoint contrasts slightly greater than in the primary analysis.

Results from selection model analyses of the primary outcome using various model parameterizations are summarized in Table 14.7. When all parameters were estimated from the data the treatment contrast was −3.10, compared with the primary result that assumed MAR of −2.16. In subsequent analyses, values for the regression parameters assessing

Table 14.5. *Results from the Primary Outcome with Data from Patients with Aberrant Residuals Excluded*

Residual Data	Number of Observations	Endpoint Contrast
All Data	1,293	−2.16
DropPlacebo	1,261	−1.94
DropDrug	1,278	−2.17
DropAll	1,246	−1.98

Table 14.6. *Results from Inclusive Modeling wGEE and MI Analyses of the Primary Outcome*

Method	Endpoint Contrast
MI	−2.26
wGEE	−2.30

the association between the current, possibly missing outcome and the probability of dropout were input across a wide range of values to determine how extreme results would have to be in order to overturn the existence of a treatment effect.

First, consider the results when input values for both psi 5 and psi 6 = 0. This result assumed MAR because the association between possibly missing efficacy outcomes and dropout was 0. As expected, the selection model results when psi 5 and psi 6 = 0 matched the primary MAR results where dropout was ignored.

Negative values for psi 5 and psi 6 indicated that as efficacy outcomes for the current, possibly missing outcome showed greater improvement, the probability patients dropped out at that visit increased, and the respective LSMEANS for the within group changes were greater than the LSMEANS from the MAR results with psi 5 and psi 6 = 0. Positive values for psi 5 and psi 6 indicated that as efficacy outcomes for the

Table 14.7. *Results from Selection Model Analyses of the Primary Outcome*

	Psi 5[1]		Psi 6[1]		Est	
	0.50	0.25	0.0	−0.25	(−0.40)	−0.50
0.50	−2.23	−2.87	−4.05	−6.32	−6.10	
0.25	−1.78	−2.18	−3.28	−4.44	−5.19	
0.0	−0.45	−1.17	−2.16	−3.22	−3.88	
Est. (−0.10)					−3.10	
−0.25	0.73	0.00	−1.10	−2.12	−2.81	
−0.50	1.48	0.74	0.42	−1.41	−2.11	

[1] Psi5 and psi 6 are the regression coefficients for placebo and drug, respectively, that the association between the current, possibly missing efficacy scores and the logit for probability of dropout. The bolded and underlined value where psi 5 and psi 6 were input as 0 corresponds to MAR.

Est = the values for psi 5 and 6 that were estimated from the data. Other values of psi 5 and psi 6 were input into the analysis

Table 14.8. *Results from Pattern-Mixture Model Analyses of the Primary Outcome*

Identifying Restriction	Endpoint Contrast
NFD_CCMV[1]	−1.88
NFD_NCMV[2]	−2.21

[1] NFD_CCMV = non future dependent complete case missing value
[2] NFD_NCNV = non future dependent neighboring case missing value

current, possibly missing outcome showed less improvement, the probability patients dropped out at that visit decreased, and the respective LSMEANS for the within group changes were less than in the MAR case.

Whenever the values for psi 5 and psi 6 were the same (underlined values on diagonal), the treatment contrast was close to the MAR result, although other aspects of the analyses, such as within-group mean changes, differed from the MAR result.

When psi 5 and psi 6 differed, treatment contrasts from the selection model differed from the primary analysis according to a consistent pattern. Whenever psi 6 (the regression coefficient for the drug treated group) was smaller than psi 5 (the regression coefficient for the placebo group) (i.e., either smaller in positive magnitude or larger in negative magnitude), the treatment contrast from the selection model was greater than from the primary analysis; when the opposite was true, the treatment contrast was smaller.

Results from pattern-mixture model analyses of the primary outcome using various identifying restrictions are summarized in Table 14.8. Using the non-future-dependent complete case missing value restriction (NFD_CCMV) yielded an endpoint contrast of −1.88, slightly smaller than the primary result of −2.16. Using the non-future-dependent neighboring case missing value restriction (NFD_NCMV) yielded an endpoint contrast of −2.21, slightly greater than the primary result. However, given that the amount of information to borrow from neighboring cases was less than from complete cases, the standard error from NFD_NCMV was also larger.

Results from shared parameter model analyses of the primary outcome are summarized in Table 14.9. Using the model that had no linkage between the dropout and measurement models yielded an endpoint contrast of −2.30. This was slightly different from the other

Table 14.9. *Results from Shared-Parameter Model Analyses of the Primary Outcome*

Model	Endpoint Contrast
Naïve model (MAR)	−2.30
Int + slope linkage	−2.19
Int + slope by trt linkage	−1.99

MAR results because of the simplified model that was necessary for the shared parameter model. Using the intercept and slope linkage yielded a slightly smaller endpoint contrast. Using separate intercept and slope linkages yielded a further slight decrease in the endpoint contrast.

Results from placebo multiple imputation analyses of the primary outcome are summarized in Table 14.10. Missing values were imputed for all patients, not just those who discontinued for adverse events. Using a restrictive imputation model yielded an endpoint contrast of −1.73. Using an inclusive imputation model that also included age and gender yielded an endpoint contrast of −1.69. The pMI results were used as a worst reasonable case MNAR analyses, forming the lower bound for the interval of plausible values.

Summary

Results from influence, correlation, and residual diagnostics are summarized in Table 14.11. Considering these results jointly fosters a clearer interpretation of the overall sensitivity of results to various aspects of the primary analysis. For residual and influence diagnostics, the range in estimates can be compared versus the results from the full data set. In assessing the impact of correlation structure, the range in results from the various models can be compared to results from the best fit model.

Table 14.10. *Results from Placebo Multiple Imputation Analyses of the Primary Outcome*

Imputation model	Endpoint Contrast
Restrictive	−1.73
Inclusive	−1.69

Table 14.11. *Summary of Results from Influence, Correlation, and Residual Diagnostics*

	Best Fit Estimate	Range in Estimates	
		Low	High
Correlation	2.16	2.08	2.32
Residual	NA	1.94	2.17
Site influence	NA	2.06	2.56
Patient influence	NA	2.20	2.75

These results showed that the magnitude of the treatment effect was not driven by a few influential patients or influential sites, and that the original choice of correlation structure was appropriate, and even if it had not been appropriate, inferences were consistent across plausible correlation structures.

Results from sensitivity analyses for missing data are summarized in Table 14.12.

In assessing the potential impact of MNAR data, treatment contrasts from the inclusive models can be compared to the primary result. For the MNAR analyses, the range in results can be compared to results from the primary analysis and results within each method can be compared to results from the MAR implementation of that method. In the efficacy context, the pMI results can form the lower bound, or worst reasonable estimate of efficacy, to be combined with other sensitivity analyses to define a "region of ignorance" – that is, a region wherein there is high

Table 14.12. *Summary of Missing Data Sensitivity Analysis Results*

Method	MAR Estimate	Range in MNAR Estimates	
		Low	High
MI_Inclusive	−2.26		
wGEE_Inclusive	−2.30		
Selection Model	−2.16		−3.10
PMM		−1.88	−2.21
SPM	−2.30	−2.00	−2.19
pMI		−1.69	−1.73

probability that the true value lies, but exactly where is not certain. Potentially, prior experience could also guide plausible values of psi 5 and psi 6 to input into the selection model. However, for the present application, prior experience was lacking and a plausible range was not predetermined. Hence, inference from the selection model is based on only the best fit estimate of a −3.10 endpoint contrast. The endpoint contrasts across the various MNAR analyses ranged from approximately −1.7 as the worst reasonable case estimate via pMI to the −3.1 result from the selection model. Most of the estimates from the various approaches were close to the estimate from the primary analysis. These results suggested that the significant result from the primary analysis was not likely biased in favor of the treatment to an important degree by MNAR data. Specifically, these results support the conclusion that the primary result was robust to bias from MNAR data.

When using the pMI result to assess the secondary objective of effectiveness, the result of a treatment advantage of 1.7 was approximately 80% the magnitude of the primary result that assessed efficacy. In other words, the effectiveness of the drug was approximately 80% as great as the efficacy that would have been achieved if all patients stayed in the trial.

14.6 Considerations

In the example data, no evidence was found for appreciable influence of individual observations (residuals) or that results were markedly swayed by influential patients or sites. Little evidence for exaggerated estimates of the treatment effect resulting from MNAR data was found as results from inclusive MAR models, and a variety of MNAR models were consistent with the primary likelihood-based result that assumed MAR.

The pMI results set a useful lower bound of plausibility when interpreted in a worst reasonable case MNAR efficacy context. When viewed in an effectiveness context, the pMI results suggested that 80% of the theoretical efficacy that would have been achieved had all patients stayed in the trial was actually obtained in this sample of patients, some of whom completed the trial and some of whom discontinued early.

Putting Principles into Practice

15.1 Introduction

Missing data is an ever-present problem in clinical trials, which can destroy the balance provided by randomization and thereby bias treatment group comparisons. Data simulation has provided a powerful platform for comparing how well analytic methods perform with incomplete data. In contrast, methods of preventing missing data cannot be evaluated via simulation and actual clinical trials are not designed to assess factors that influence retention. Therefore, many confounding factors can mask or exaggerate differences in rates of missing data attributable to trial methods. Not surprisingly then, the literature contains more information on how to treat missing data than on how to prevent it.

In order to understand the potential impact of missing data and to choose an appropriate analysis, the mechanism(s) leading to the missingness must be considered. In longitudinal clinical trials, MCAR is not likely to hold, MAR is often plausible but never testable, and going beyond MAR to MNAR requires assumptions that are also not testable. Although some analyses are better than others in mitigating the problems caused by missing data, no analysis *solves* the problems. Even if bias is minimized, the loss of information can still be considerable.

A useful by-product of the debates on analytic approaches for incomplete data has been consideration of primary estimands. Issues regarding choice of estimand center on whether interest is in the effects of the drug if taken as directed (de jure hypothesis) or in effects of the drug as actually taken (de facto hypothesis). Clarity on the objectives is critical because choice of estimand influences the design and analysis of the trial.

15.2 Prevention

Given the analytic limitations, the best approach to dealing with missing data is to prevent it. Hence, the NRC expert panel on treating and preventing missing data concluded maximizing the number of participants who are maintained on the protocol-specified interventions until the outcome data are collected is the most important factor in mitigating the impact of missing data (NRC, 2010).

In addition to scarce evidence on design approaches to minimize missing data, design options often entail trade-offs. A design feature that reduces the probability of dropout is likely to have consequences in other aspects of the trial. For example, an enrichment design may lower dropout, but this requires that a subset with more favorable benefit-risk can be readily and rapidly identified in a trial, and the inferential focus is on the enriched subset, not all patients. Flexible dosing may also limit early discontinuations, but it cannot be used in trials where inference about specific doses is required, such as dose response studies.

Consider the data used for the analytic example in Chapter 14. The rates of early discontinuation were about 40% for the experimental drug and 35% for placebo. Assume the NRC (NRC, 2010) recommendation of specifying a minimum rate of completion is followed and that the goal for a subsequent trial is to have no more than 20% dropout. What can be done to achieve this goal in the subsequent trial?

In the example trial, each treatment arm had approximately 17% of patients discontinue early for either lack of efficacy or adverse events. Thus, more than half the early discontinuations were for reasons not directly attributable to the causal effects of the drug.

Assume an enrichment strategy and greater flexibility in dosing are planned for the subsequent trial. Although these approaches may help reduce dropout for the drug group, it is unclear what if any impact there would be on the placebo group. Hence, consider only the drug group for now.

Of course, how much these design options may help is only speculation. But reducing early attrition attributable to efficacy and tolerability by half via design changes would be meaningful. In the example data, doing so would have reduced total dropout in the drug group by about

9% (17%/2), from about 40% to 31%. Even eliminating all dropouts attributable to adverse events and lack of efficacy would fall short of the 20% dropout goal.

Reasons for dropout other than adverse events and lack of efficacy can include patient decision, physician decision, protocol violation, and loss to follow-up. These reasons leave doubt about treatment-related causality and the impact these missing data may have on treatment comparisons. The ideal trial may be one in which the only reasons for discontinuing the initially randomized study drug are lack of efficacy, adverse events, and withdrawal of consent. Depending on the goals of the study, follow-up data after discontinuation of the initial study drug and/or initiation of rescue medications might be collected.

To achieve such disposition results, proper processes, case report forms, informed consents, data capture procedures, minimal patient burden, patient accommodations, and other measures need to be in place. However, trial sponsors, sites, and patients also need to believe in the importance of complete data. Rigorous selection of sites and patients, combined with education, monitoring, and incentives, can help in this regard.

Simply put, lowering rates of dropout can be as much about behavior as design and process. If completion rates are focused on as much as enrollment rates, considerable progress may be possible. Importantly, changing attitudes and behaviors regarding missing data will likely help increase retention in drug groups and control groups, whereas enrichment designs, flexible dosing, and other design features may have greater impact on drug groups than on the placebo groups.

It is also important to recognize that minimizing loss to follow-up in essence reduces the potential for MNAR data. Consider a patient that had been doing well, but then relapsed into a worsened condition at Week 6 of a 12-week trial and discontinued. If the Week 6 observation reflecting the worsened condition was obtained, the missingness mechanism could be MAR. However, if the patient was lost to follow-up and there was no Week 6 observation, only Weeks 1–5 that reflected the favorable outcomes, the missingness would be MNAR. Trials should therefore make extensive efforts to minimize loss to follow-up, and thereby ensure that the patients who discontinue the originally randomized medications do so for reasons that are causally related to the study medications, and that those reasons are captured in the data.

Success in these efforts would result in completion rates that were as high as possible given the drug(s) being studied, and what missing data did exist would arise from an MAR mechanism, thereby fostering formulation of sensible analyses.

15.3 Analysis

Despite all efforts to minimize missing data, anticipating complete data is not realistic.

Consensus is emerging that a primary analysis based on MAR is often reasonable. Such an approach would be especially reasonable when combined with rigorous efforts to maximize the number of patients retained on the initially randomized medications and minimizing loss to follow-up. Nevertheless, appropriateness of any analysis plan will also hinge on clarity of the primary estimand and on sensitivity analyses to assess robustness of inferences to missing data assumptions.

Within the MAR framework, likelihood-based analyses, multiple imputation, and weighted GEE are all well-studied methods. The specific attributes of each method can be used to tailor an analysis to the situation at hand. With an MAR primary analysis in place, assessing robustness of conclusions to departures from MAR is critical.

Although consensus does not exist on how to draw inferences in a sensitivity framework, recent guidance clarifies a number of principles. First, although there may be need for additional sensitivity analyses inspired by trial results, a parsimonious set of plausible sensitivity analyses should be prespecified and reported. Results from these prespecified analyses form the basis for assessing uncertainty in inference attributable to untestable assumptions regarding missing data. Justification for the chosen set of sensitivity analyses can be guided by previous experience. The most relevant information for choosing sensitivity analyses would be previous trials of the same drug in the same disease. However, general experience across the therapeutic area, perhaps obtained from retrospective analyses, can also be useful.

Whenever the primary analysis assumes MAR, a significant focus of sensitivity analyses will include MNAR methods to assess how departures from MAR may have influenced inferences. Three most common families of MNAR analyses include shared-parameter models, pattern mixture models, and selection models. Controlled imputation approaches have not been as thoroughly explored in the literature and have only recently been used in practice. However, they may prove particularly useful in sensitivity analyses. In many situations, controlled imputation can be used to construct a principled set of imputations that exhibit a specific statistical behavior useful in sensitivity analyses. For example, a worst reasonable case may be constructed by assuming the values of drug-treated patients take on the characteristics of the control group after discontinuation or initiation of rescue meds. This result can then be used to define the lower bound of plausible values for the set of sensitivity analyses. Alternatively, the imputations can be controlled in some manner to provide a progressively more severe stress test to assess how extreme results would need to be to overturn the primary result.

15.4 Software

By itself, a road map gets one nowhere. A vehicle is needed. For the analytic road map, that vehicle is software. The environment in which medical interventions are developed puts a premium on standardized, validated software. Regulators and sponsors require validated algorithms and programs to be certain that the intended analyses are implemented correctly. Without adequate software tools, complex programs such as those to conduct MNAR analyses are extremely difficult and time consuming to develop and validate.

The NRC expert panel on the prevention and treatment of missing data noted the need for specialized software tools as an important area for further work. Simply put, without better software tools, sensitivity analyses in general and MNAR analyses in particular will be difficult to implement and these difficulties will limit their use.

For those interested in software tools, the programs used to analyze the example data in Chapter 14 may be obtained at www.missingdata.org.uk.

The Web site provides details on these programs and how to use them, along with an example data set on which to run the programs. Although the programs used in Chapter 14 will be archived at that site, newer, more generalized versions of these programs and additional programs will be made available periodically, and users are encouraged to access the latest versions of the programs. The programs used in Chapter 14 have not had their functionality validated across broad uses. Nevertheless, these programs will hopefully serve as a useful starting point and can be modified relatively easily for alternative usages.

15.5 Concluding Thoughts

The analytic road map and other ideas regarding prevention and treatment of missing data presented in this book are not meant to be prescriptive as to exactly how trials should be designed, implemented, and analyzed. Rather, the intent has been to illustrate application of key principles that have arisen from recent guidance.

As the clinical contexts vary between studies, so too should the trial design and conduct options, along with the specific form of the sensitivity analyses. In particular, the extent of the sensitivity analyses is dictated by the diversity in assumptions that are plausible.

Reasonable measures to reduce missing data combined with appropriate analytic plans that include sensitivity analyses can markedly reduce the uncertainty in results and increase the information gained from medical research. Recent research has provided useful guidance on these various approaches, and the intent of this book has been to provide researchers with a practical guide to make use of them.

Bibliography

Aerts, M., Guys, H., Molenberghs, G. and Ryan, L. M. (2002). *Topics in Modelling of Clustered Data*. Chapman and Hall, London.

Carpenter, J. R., Kenward, M. G., and Vansteelandt, S. (2006). A comparison of multiple imputation and doubly robust estimation for analyses with missing data. *Journal of the Royal Statistical Society, Series A*, 169: 571–584.

Carpenter, J. R. and Kenward, M. G. (2007). *Missing Data in Clinical Trials: A Practical Guide*. Birmingham: National Health Service Coordinating.

Centre for Research Methodology. (2009). Online at: http://www.pcpoh.bham.ac.uk/publichealth/methodology/projects/RM03 JH17 MK.shtml (accessed May 28, 2009).

Cnaan, A., Laird, N. M., and Slasor, P. (1997). Using the general linear mixed model to analyse unbalanced repeated measures and longitudinal data. *Statistics in Medicine*, 16 (20): 2349–2380.

Cohen, J. (1992). A power primer. *Psychological Bulletin*, 112: 155–159.

Collins, L. M., Schafer, J. L., and Kam, C. M. (2001). A comparison of inclusive and restrictive strategies in modern missing data procedures. *Psychology Methods*, 6 (4): 330–351.

Committee for Medicinal Products for Human Use (CHMP). (2010). Guideline on missing data in confirmatory clinical trials. EMA/CPMP/EWP/1776/99 Rev. 1.

Cook, R. D., and Weisberg, S. (1982). *Residuals and Influence in Regression*. New York: Chapman & Hall.

Copas, J. B., and Li, H. G. (1997). Inference for non-random samples (with discussion). *Journal of the Royal Statistical Society B*, 59: 55–96.

Detke, M. J., Lu, Y., Goldstein, D. J., McNamara, R. K., and Demitrack, M. A. (2002). Duloxetine 60 mg once daily dosing versus placebo in the acute treatment of major depression. *Journal of Psychiatric Research*, 36: 383–390.

Diggle, P. D., and Kenward, M. G. (1994). Informative dropout in longitudinal data analysis (with discussion). *Applied Statistics*, 43: 49–93.

Diggle, P. J., Heagerty, P., Liang K. Y., and Seger, S. L. (2002). *The Analysis of Longitudinal Data*, 2nd Edition. Oxford: Oxford University Press.

Draper D. (1995). Assessment and propagation of model uncertainty (with discussion). *Journal of the Royal Statistical Society B*, 57: 45.

Fahrmeir, L., and Tutz, G. (2001). *Multivariate Statistical Modelling Based on Generalized Linear Models*. Heidelberg: Springer.

Fitzmaurice, G. M., Laird, N. M., and Ware, J. H. (2004). *Applied Longitudinal Analysis*. Hoboken, NJ: Wiley Interscience.

Fedorov, V. V., and Liu, T. 2007. Enrichment design. *Wiley Encyclopedia of Clinical Trials*, 1–8.

Fleming, T. R. (2011). Addressing missing data in clinical trials. *Annals of Internal Medicine*, 154: 113–117.

Hamilton M: A rating scale for depression. *J Neurol Neurosurg Psychiatry* 1960, 23: 56–61.

Harville, David A. (1977). Maximum likelihood approaches to variance component estimation and to related problems. *Journal of the American Statistical Association*, 72 (358): 320–338.

Hogan, J. W., and Laird, N. M. (1997). Mixture models for the joint distribution of repeated measures and event times. *Statistics in Medicine*, 16: 239–258.

Horvitz, D. G., and Thompson D. J. (1952). A generalization of sampling without replacement from a finite universe. *Journal of the American Statistical Association*, 47: 663–685.

ICH guidelines. Online at: http://www.ich.org/cache/compo/276–254-1.html

Jansen, I., Beunckens, C., Molenberghs, G., Verbeke, G., Mallinckrodt, C. H. (2006a). Analyzing incomplete binary longitudinal clinical trial data. *Statistical Science*, 21 (1): 52–69.

Jansen, I., Hens, N., Molenberghs, G., Aerts, M., Verbeke, G., and Kenward, M. G. (2006b). The nature of sensitivity in missing not at random models. *Computational Statistics and Data Analysis*, 50: 830–858.

Kenward, M. G. (1998). Selection models for repeated measurements with non-random dropout: an illustration of sensitivity. *Statistics in Medicine*, 17 (23): 2723–2732.

Kim, Y. (2011). Missing data handling in chronic pain trials. *Journal of Biopharmaceutical Statistics*, 21 (2): 311–325.

Landin, R., DeBrota, D. J., DeVries, T. A., Potter, W. Z., and Demitrack, M. A. (2000). The impact of restrictive entry criterion during the placebo lead-in period. *Biometrics*, 56 (1): 271–278.

Laird, N. M., and Ware, J. H. (1982). Random-effects models for longitudinal data. *Biometrics*, 38 (4): 963–974.

Laird, N. M. (1994). Informative dropout in longitudinal data analysis. *Applied Statistics*, 43: 84.

Leon, A. C., Hakan, D., and Hedeken, D. (2007). Bias reduction with an adjustment for participants' intent to drop out of a randomized controlled clinical trial. *Clinical Trials*, 4: 540–547.

Liang, K. Y., and Zeger, S. (1986). Longitudinal data analysis using generalized linear models. *Biometrika*, 73 (1): 13–22.

Liang, K. Y., and Zeger, S. (2000). Longitudinal data analysis of continuous and discrete responses for pre-post designs. *Sankhya: The Indian Journal of Statistics*, 62 (Series B): 134–148.

Lipkovich, I., Duan, Y., and Ahmed, S. (2005). Multiple imputation compared with restricted pseudo-likelihood and generalized estimating equations for analysis of binary repeated measures in clinical studies. *Pharmaceutical Statistics*, 4 (4): 267–285.

Little, R. J. A. (1993). Pattern-mixture models for multivariate incomplete data. *Journal of American Statistical Association*, 88 (421): 125–134.

Little, R. J. A. (1994). A class of pattern-mixture models for normal incomplete data. *Biometrika*, 81 (3): 471–483.

Little, R. J. A. (1995). Modeling the drop-out mechanism in repeated measures studies. *Journal of American Statistical Association*, 90 (431): 1112–1121.

Little, R. J. A., and Rubin, D. B. (2002). *Statistical Analysis with Missing Data*, 2nd Edition. New York: Wiley.

Little, R., and Yau, L. (1996). Intent-to-treat analysis for longitudinal studies with drop-outs. *Biometrics*, 52 (4): 1324–1333.

Little, R. J. A., and Yau, L. (1998). Statistical techniques for analyzing data from prevention trials: Treatment of no-shows using Rubin's causal model. *Psychological Methods*, 3: 147–159.

Liu, G., and Gould, A. L. (2002). Comparison of alternative strategies for analysis of longitudinal trials with dropouts. *Journal of Biopharmaceutical Statistics*, 12 (2): 207–226.

Lu, K., and Mehrotra, D. (2009). Specification of covariance structure in longitudinal data analysis for randomized clinical trials. *Statistics in Medicine*, 4: 474–488.

Ma, G., Troxel, A. B., and Heitjan, D. F. (2005). An index of local sensitivity to nonignorable drop-out in longitudinal modeling. *Statistics in Medicine*, 24 (14): 2129–2150.

Mallinckrodt, C. H., Clark, S. W., Carroll, R. J., and Molenberghs, G. (2003). Assessing response profiles from incomplete longitudinal clinical trial data under regulatory considerations. *Journal of Biopharmaceutical Statistics*, 13 (2): 179–190.

Mallinckrodt, C. H., Kaiser, C. J., Watkin, J. G., Molenberghs, G., and Carroll, R. J. (2004). The effect of correlation structure on treatment contrasts estimated from incomplete clinical trial data with likelihood-based repeated measures compared with last observation carried forward ANOVA. *Clinical Trials*, 1 (6): 477–489.

Mallinckrodt, C. H., and Kenward, M. G. (2009). Conceptual considerations regarding choice of endpoints, hypotheses, and analyses in longitudinal clinical trials. *Drug Information Journal*, 43 (4): 449–458.

Mallinckrodt, C. H., Lane, P. W., Schnell, D., Peng, Y., and Mancuso, J. P. (2008). Recommendations for the primary analysis of continuous endpoints in longitudinal clinical trials. *Drug Information Journal*, 42: 305–319.

Mallinckrodt, C. H., Lin, Q., Lipkovich, I., and Molenberghs, G. (forthcoming). A structured approach to choosing estimands and estimators in longitudinal clinical trials. *Pharmaceutical Statistics*, (In Press).

Mallinckrodt, C. H., Tamura, R. N., and Tanaka, Y. (2011). Improving signal detection and reducing placebo response in psychiatric clinical trials. *Journal of Psychiatric Research*, 45: 1202–1207.

McCullagh, P. and Nelder, J. A. (1989) *Generalized Linear Models*. London: Chapman & Hall.

Meng, X.-L. (1994). Multiple-imputation inferences with uncongenial sources of input. *Statistical Science*, 9: 538–558.

Molenberghs, G., and Kenward, M. G. (2007). *Missing Data in Clinical Studies*. Chichester: John Wiley & Sons.

Molenberghs, G., Kenward, M. G., and Lesaffre, E. (1997). The analysis of longitudinal ordinal data with nonrandom dropout. *Biometrika*, 84 (1): 33–44.

Molenberghs, G., Thijs, H., Jansen, I., Beunckens, C., Kenward, M. G., Mallinckrodt, C., and Carroll, R. J. (2004). Analyzing incomplete longitudinal clinical trial data. *Biostatistics*, 5 (3): 445–464.

Molenberghs, G., and Verbeke, G. (2005). *Models for Discrete Longitudinal Data*. New York: Springer.

Molenberghs, G., Verbeke, G., Thijs, H., Lesaffre, E., and Kenward, M. (2001). Mastitis in dairy cattle: Local influence to assess sensitivity of the dropout process. *Computational Statistics & Data Analysis*, 37 (1): 93–113.

National Research Council (2010). *The Prevention and Treatment of Missing Data in Clinical Trials. Panel on Handling Missing Data in Clinical Trials*. Committee on National Statistics, Division of Behavioral and Social Sciences and Education. Washington, DC: The National Academies Press.

O'Neill, R. T., and Temple, R. (2012). The prevention and treatment of missing data in clinical trials: An FDA perspective on the importance of dealing with it. *Clinical Pharmacology and Therapeutics*. doi:10.1038/clpt.2011.340.

Permutt T and Pinheiro J. (2009). Dealing with the missing data challenge in clinical trials. *Drug Information Journal*. 43: 403–408.

Ratitch B, O'Kelly M. Implementation of Pattern-Mixture Models Using Standard SAS/STAT Procedures. *PharmaSUG* 2011. Available at http://pharmasug.org/proceedings/2011/SP/PharmaSUG-2011-SP04.pdf (accessed October 4, 2011).

Robins, J. M., Rotnizky, A., and Zhao, L. P. (1994). Estimation of regression coefficients when some regressors are not always observed. *Journal of the American Statistical Association*, 89: 846–866.

Robins, J. M., Rotnitzky, A., and Zhao, L. P. (1995). Analysis of semi-parametric regression models for repeated outcomes in the presence of missing data. *Journal of the American Statistical Association*, 90: 106–121.

Rubin, D. B. (1976). Inference and missing data. *Biometrika*, 63 (3): 581–592.

Rubin, D. B. (1978). Multiple imputations in sample surveys – a phenomenological Bayesian approach to nonresponse. In *Imputation and Editing of Faulty or Missing Survey Data*. Washington, DC: U.S. Department of Commerce, pp. 1–23.

Rubin, D. B. (1987). *Multiple Imputation for Nonresponse in Surveys*. New York: John Wiley & Sons.

Rubin, D. B. (1994). Informative dropout in longitudinal data analysis. *Applied Statistics*, 43: 80–82.

SAS Institute Inc. (2003). SAS/STAT® User's Guide, Version 9.1, Cary, NC: SAS Institute, Inc.

Schafer, J. (2003). Multiple imputation in multivariate problems when the imputation and analysis models differ. *Statistics Neerlandica*, 57: 19–35.

Shen, S., Beunckens, C., Mallinckrodt, C., and Molenberghs, G. (2006). A local influence sensitivity analysis for incomplete longitudinal depression data. *Journal of Biopharmacological Statistics*, 16 (3): 365–384.

Shen, J., Kobak, K. A., Zhao, Y., Alexander, M., and Kane, J. (2008). Use of remote centralized raters via live 2-way video in a multi central clinical trial for schizophrenia. *Journal of Clinical Psychopharmacology*, 28 (6): 691–693.

Siddiqui, O., Hung, H. M., and O'Neill, R. O. (2009). MMRM vs. LOCF: A comprehensive comparison based on simulation study and 25 NDA datasets. *Journal of Biopharmaceutical Statistics*, 19 (2): 227–246.

Snedecor, G. W., and Cochran, W. G. (1989). Statistical Methods. 8th edition. Aimes: Iowa State University Press.

Temple, R. (2005). Enrichment designs: Efficiency in development of cancer treatments. *Journal of Clinical Oncology*, 23 (22): 4838–4839.

Teshome, B., Lipkovich, I., Molenberghs, G., and Mallinckrodt, C. (forthcoming). A multiple imputation based approach to sensitivity analyses and effectiveness assessments in longitudinal clinical trials. *Journal of Biopharmacological Statistics.*

Thijs, H., Molenberghs, G., Michiels, B., Verbeke, G., and Curran, D. (2002) Strategies to fit pattern-mixture models. *Biostatistics*, 3: 245–265.

Thijs, H., Molenberghs, G., and Verbeke G. (2000). The milk protein trial: Influence analysis of the dropout process. *Biomedical Journal*, 42 (5): 617–646.

Troxel, A. B., Ma, G., and Heitjan, D. F. (2004). An index of local sensitivity to nonignorability. *Statistica Sinica*, 14: 1221–1237.

Tsiatis, A. A. (2006). *Semiparametric Theory and Missing Data.* New York: Springer.

Verbeke, G., and Molenberghs, G. (2000). *Linear Mixed Models for Longitudinal Data.* New York: Springer.

Verbeke, G., Molenberghs, G., Thijs, H., Lesaffre, E., and Kenward, M. G. (2001). Sensitivity analysis for nonrandom dropout: a local influence approach. *Biometrics*, 57 (1): 7–14.

Wonnacott, T. H., and Wonnacott, R. J. (1981). *Regression: A Second Course in Statistics.* New York: Wiley.

Wu, M. C., and Carroll, R. J. (1988). Estimation and comparison of changes in the presence of informative right censoring by modeling the censoring process. *Biometrics*, 44: 175–188.

Wu, M. C., and Bailey, K. R. (1989). Estimation and comparison of changes in the presence of informative right censoring: conditional linear model. *Biometrics*, 45 (3): 939–955.

Zhu, H. T., and Lee, S. Y. (2001). Local influence for incomplete-data models. *Journal of the Royal Statistical Society B*, 63: 111–126.

Index